STUDENT WORKBOOK TO ACCOMPANY

INTRODUCTION TO MEDICAL TERMINOLOGY

Third Edition

Ann Ehrlich
Carol L. Schroeder

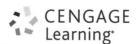
CENGAGE
Learning·

Australia · Brazil · Japan · Korea · Mexico · Singapore · Spain · United Kingdom · United States

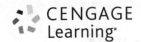

CENGAGE
Learning

Student Workbook to Accompany
Introduction to Medical Terminology,
Third Edition
Ann Ehrlich and Carol L. Schroeder

Senior Vice President/General Manager, Skills and Product Planning: Dawn Gerrain

Product Director, Health Care Skills: Stephen Helba

Product Team Manager: Matthew Seeley

Senior Director, Development: Marah Bellegarde

Product Development Manager, Health Care Skills: Juliet Steiner

Senior Content Developer, Health Care Skills: Debra M. Myette-Flis

Product Assistant: Jennifer Wheaton

Marketing Brand Manager: Wendy Mapstone

Senior Production Director: Wendy Troeger

Production Manager: Andrew Crouth

Content Project Manager: Thomas Heffernan

Senior Art Director: Jack Pendleton

Cover image(s): iStock.com/Vetta Collection/ commotion_design, www.Shutterstock.com/ super1973

For product information and technology assistance, contact us at
Cengage Learning Customer & Sales Support, 1-800-354-9706
For permission to use material from this text or product,
submit all requests online at **www.cengage.com/permissions**.
Further permissions questions can be e-mailed to
permissionrequest@cengage.com

Library of Congress Control Number: 2013932313

ISBN-13: 978-1-133-95173-5

ISBN-10: 1-133-95173-2

Cengage Learning
200 First Stamford Place, 4th Floor
Stamford, CT 06902
USA

Cengage Learning is a leading provider of customized learning solutions with office locations around the globe, including Singapore, the United Kingdom, Australia, Mexico, Brazil, and Japan. Locate your local office at: **www.cengage.com/global**

Cengage Learning products are represented in Canada by Nelson Education, Ltd.

To learn more about Cengage Learning, visit **www.cengage.com**

Purchase any of our products at your local college store or at our preferred online store **www.cengagebrain.com**

Notice to the Reader
Publisher does not warrant or guarantee any of the products described herein or perform any independent analysis in connection with any of the product information contained herein. Publisher does not assume, and expressly disclaims, any obligation to obtain and include information other than that provided to it by the manufacturer. The reader is expressly warned to consider and adopt all safety precautions that might be indicated by the activities described herein and to avoid all potential hazards. By following the instructions contained herein, the reader willingly assumes all risks in connection with such instructions. The publisher makes no representations or warranties of any kind, including but not limited to, the warranties of fitness for particular purpose or merchantability, nor are any such representations implied with respect to the material set forth herein, and the publisher takes no responsibility with respect to such material. The publisher shall not be liable for any special, consequential, or exemplary damages resulting, in whole or part, from the readers' use of, or reliance upon, this material.

Printed in the United States of America
7 8 9 10 11 12   22 21 20 19 18

C O N T E N T S

Preface   iv

Chapter   1: Introduction to Medical Terminology   1
Chapter   2: The Human Body in Health and Disease   9
                    Word Part Review   17
Chapter   3: The Skeletal System   23
Chapter   4: The Muscular System   31
Chapter   5: The Cardiovascular System   39
Chapter   6: The Lymphatic and Immune Systems   47
Chapter   7: The Respiratory System   55
Chapter   8: The Digestive System   63
Chapter   9: The Urinary System   71
Chapter 10: The Nervous System   79
Chapter 11: Special Senses: The Eyes and Ears   87
Chapter 12: Skin: The Integumentary System   95
Chapter 13: The Endocrine System   103
Chapter 14: The Reproductive Systems   111
Chapter 15: Diagnostic Procedures, Nuclear Medicine,
                    and Pharmacology   119

                    Comprehensive Medical Terminology Review   127
                    Flash Cards   155

PREFACE

To the Student

Welcome to the *Student Workbook to Accompany Introduction to Medical Terminology*, Third Edition. This workbook contains many features to make your mastery of medical terminology easier, and it would be to your benefit to take advantage of them.

Using this Workbook

Chapter Features

There is a chapter in this workbook to accompany each chapter in your textbook. Each workbook chapter contains 100 Learning Exercises. To make these activities more interesting and challenging, they are in a variety of formats. With each question, there is a space for you to write your answer in the workbook. After you complete the exercises, follow your teacher's instructions for handing in your work and having it corrected. When these pages are returned to you, save them in your notebook for use as an additional review resource.

Writing the answer to each question rather than just circling a letter reinforces the material you are learning. Many questions include a variety of answer choices, and you'll be pleasantly surprised at how quickly you can complete the exercises!

The Learning Exercises for each chapter include:

- Matching Word Parts
- Definitions
- Matching Structures, Conditions or Techniques
- Which Word?
- Spelling Counts
- Matching Abbreviations, Conditions or Diseases
- Term Selection
- Sentence Completion
- True/False
- Clinical Conditions
- Which Is the Correct Medical Term
- Challenge Word Building
- Labeling

Word Part Review

There is a Word Part Review section to be completed after you have studied Chapters 1 and 2. This short section provides additional practice in working with word parts, plus a test to evaluate how well you've mastered their use.

Because most medical terms are based on word parts, mastery of these components is very important before you begin your study of the body systems. If you have trouble here, this is the time to ask for help!

Comprehensive Review

At the end of your workbook there is a Comprehensive Medical Terminology Review section. This contains study tips, review questions, and a simulated final test, all of which are designed to help you prepare for your final examination; however, be aware that none of the simulated final test questions are from the actual final test. You'll find this section very helpful when you use it on your own or in conjunction with class review sessions.

Flash Cards

The activity card pages at the back of this workbook are designed to be removed and used as flash cards. Flash cards are a great study aid, and early in your course you'll want to follow the instructions for removing these pages, separating the cards, and using them in a variety of fun study activities.

Good Luck!

It is our hope that your study of medical terminology will be interesting and rewarding. We also hope that the *Introduction to Medical Terminology* text and this workbook help you find a career in health care that will bring you professional success and satisfaction.

Ann Ehrlich
Carol L. Schroeder

CHAPTER 1

Introduction to Medical Terminology

Learning Exercises

Class _____   Name _____

Matching Word Parts 1

Write the correct answer in the middle column.

Definition	Correct Answer	Possible Answers
1.1. bad, difficult, painful	_____	**-algia**
1.2. excessive, increased	_____	**dys-**
1.3. enlargement	_____	**-ectomy**
1.4. pain, suffering	_____	**-megaly**
1.5. surgical removal	_____	**hyper-**

Matching Word Parts 2

Write the correct answer in the middle column.

Definition	Correct Answer	Possible Answers
1.6. abnormal condition or disease	_____	**hypo-**
1.7. abnormal softening	_____	**-itis**
1.8. deficient, decreased	_____	**-malacia**
1.9. inflammation	_____	**-necrosis**
1.10. tissue death	_____	**-osis**

Matching Word Parts 3

Write the correct answer in the middle column.

Definition	Correct Answer	Possible Answers
1.11. bleeding, bursting forth	_____	**-ostomy**
1.12. surgical creation of an artificial opening to the body surface	_____	**-otomy**
1.13. surgical incision	_____	**-plasty**
1.14. surgical repair	_____	**-rrhage**
1.15. surgical suturing	_____	**-rrhaphy**

Matching Word Parts 4

Write the correct answer in the middle column.

Definition	Correct Answer	Possible Answers
1.16. visual examination	_____	**-rrhea**
1.17. rupture	_____	**-rrhexis**
1.18. abnormal narrowing	_____	**-sclerosis**
1.19. abnormal hardening	_____	**-scopy**
1.20. flow or discharge	_____	**-stenosis**

Definitions

Select the correct answer, and write it on the line provided.

1.21. The term _____ describes any pathologic change or disease in the spinal cord.

    myelopathy   myopathy   pyelitis   pyrosis

1.22. The medical term for higher-than-normal blood pressure is _____.

    hepatomegaly   hypertension   hypotension   supination

1.23. The term _____ means pertaining to birth.

    natal   perinatal   postnatal   prenatal

1.24. Pain is classified as a _____.

    diagnosis   sign   symptom   syndrome

1.25. In the term *myopathy*, the suffix **-pathy** means _____.

    abnormal condition   disease   inflammation   swelling

Matching Terms and Definitions 1

Write the correct answer in the middle column.

Definition	Correct Answer	Possible Answers
1.26. white blood cell	_____	acute
1.27. prediction of the probable course and outcome of a disorder	_____	edema
1.28. swelling caused by an abnormal accumulation of fluid in cells, tissues, or cavities of the body	_____	leukocyte
1.29. rapid onset	_____	prognosis
1.30. turning the palm of the hand upward	_____	supination

Matching Terms and Definitions 2

Write the correct answer in the middle column.

Definition	Correct Answer	Possible Answers
1.31. examination procedure	_____	laceration
1.32. fluid, such as pus, that leaks out of an infected wound	_____	lesion
1.33. pathologic tissue change	_____	palpitation
1.34. pounding heart	_____	palpation
1.35. torn or jagged wound, or an accidental cut wound	_____	exudate

Which Word?

Select the correct answer, and write it on the line provided.

1.36. The medical term _____ describes an inflammation of the stomach.

gastritis   gastrosis

1.37. The formation of pus is called _____.

supination   suppuration

1.38. The term meaning wound or injury is _____.

trauma   triage

1.39. The term _____ means pertaining to a virus.

viral   virile

1.40. An _____ is the surgical removal of the appendix.

appendectomy   appendicitis

Spelling Counts

Find the misspelled word in each sentence. Then write that word, spelled correctly, on the line provided.

1.41. A disease named for the person who discovered it is known as an enaponym. _____

1.42. A localized response to injury or tissue destruction is called inflimmation. _____

1.43. A fisure of the skin is a groove or crack-like sore of the skin. _____

1.44. The medical term meaning suturing together the ends of a severed nerve is neurorraphy.

_____

1.45. The medical term meaning inflammation of the tonsils is tonsilitis. _____

Matching Terms

Write the correct answer in the middle column.

Definition	Correct Answer	Possible Answers
1.46. abnormal condition or disease of the stomach	_____	syndrome
1.47. a set of signs and symptoms	_____	gastralgia
1.48. rupture of a muscle	_____	gastrosis
1.49. stomach pain	_____	pyoderma
1.50. any acute, inflammatory, pus-forming bacterial skin infection	_____	myorrhexis

Term Selection

Select the correct answer, and write it on the line provided.

1.51. The abnormal hardening of the walls of an artery or arteries is called _____.

| arteriosclerosis | arteriostenosis | arthrostenosis | atherosclerosis |

1.52. A fever is considered to be a _____.

| prognosis | sign | symptom | syndrome |

1.53. An inflammation of the stomach and small intestine is known as _____.

| gastralgia | gastroenteritis | gastritis | gastrosis |

1.54. The term meaning pain in a joint or joints is _____.

| arthralgia | arthritis | arthrocentesis | atherosclerosis |

1.55. A _____ is a physician who specializes in diagnosing and treating diseases and disorders of the skin.

| dermatologist | dermatology | neurologist | neurology |

Sentence Completion

Write the correct term on the line provided.

1.56. Lower-than-normal blood pressure is called _____.

1.57. The process of recording a radiographic study of the blood vessels after the injection of a contrast medium is known as _____.

1.58. The term meaning above or outside the ribs is _____.

1.59. A/An _____ diagnosis is also known as a rule out.

1.60. A/An _____ is an abnormal passage, usually between two internal organs or leading from an organ to the surface of the body.

True/False

If the statement is true, write **True** on the line. If the statement is false, write **False** on the line.

1.61. _____ An erythrocyte is commonly known as a red blood cell.

1.62. _____ Arteriomalacia is abnormal hardening of blood vessels of the walls of an artery or arteries.

1.63. _____ A colostomy is the surgical creation of an artificial opening between the colon and the body surface.

1.64. _____ Malaise is often the first symptom of inflammation.

1.65. _____ An infection is the invasion of the body by a disease-producing organism.

Word Surgery

Divide each term into its component word parts. Write these word parts, in sequence, on the lines provided. When necessary, use a slash (/) to indicate a combining vowel. (You may not need all of the lines provided.)

1.66. **Otorhinolaryngology** is the study of the ears, nose, and throat.

_____   _____   _____   _____

1.67. The term **mycosis** means any abnormal condition or disease caused by a fungus.

_____   _____   _____   _____

1.68. **Poliomyelitis** is a viral infection of the gray matter of the spinal cord.

_____   _____   _____   _____

1.69. **Neonatology** is the study of disorders of the newborn.

_____   _____   _____   _____

1.70. The term **endarterial** means pertaining to the interior or lining of an artery.

_____   _____   _____   _____

Clinical Conditions

Write the correct answer on the line provided.

1.71. Miguel required a/an _____ injection. This term means that the medication was placed directly within the muscle.

1.72. Mrs. Tillson underwent _____ to remove excess fluid from her abdomen.

1.73. The term *laser* is a/an _____. This means that it is a word formed from the initial letters of the major parts of a compound term.

1.74. In an accident, Felipe Valladares broke several bones in his fingers. The medical term for these injuries is fractured _____.

1.75. In case of a major disaster Cheng Lee, who is a trained paramedic, helps perform _____. This is the screening of patients to determine their relative priority of need and the proper place of treatment.

1.76. Gina's physician ordered laboratory tests that would enable him to establish a differential _____ to identify the cause of her signs and symptoms.

1.77. Jennifer plans to go to graduate school so she can specialize in _____. This specialty is concerned with the study of all aspects of diseases.

1.78. John Randolph's cancer went into _____. Although this is not a cure, his symptoms disappeared and he felt much better.

1.79. Mr. Jankowski describes that uncomfortable feeling as heartburn. The medical term for this condition is _____.

1.80. Phyllis was having great fun traveling until she ate some contaminated food and developed _____. She felt miserable and needed to stay in her hotel because of the frequent flow of loose or watery stools.

Which Is the Correct Medical Term?

Select the correct answer, and write it on the line provided.

1.81. The term _____ describes the surgical repair of a nerve.

neuralgia   neurorrhaphy   neurology   neuroplasty

1.82. The term _____ means loss of a large amount of blood in a short time.

diarrhea   hemorrhage   hepatorrhagia   otorrhagia

1.83. The term _____ means the tissue death of an artery or arteries.

arteriomalacia   arterionecrosis   arteriosclerosis   arteriostenosis

1.84. The term _____ means between, but not within, the parts of a tissue.

interstitial   intrastitial   intermuscular   intramuscular

1.85. The term _____ means enlargement of the liver.

hepatitis   hepatomegaly   nephromegaly   nephritis

Challenge Word Building

These terms are *not* found in this chapter; however, they are made up of the following familiar word parts. If you need help in creating the term, refer to your medical dictionary.

neo- = new	**arteri/o** = artery	**-algia** = pain and suffering
	arthr/o = joint	**-itis** = inflammation
	cardi/o = heart	**-ologist** = specialist
	nat/o = birth	**-otomy** = a surgical incision
	neur/o = nerve	**-rrhea** = flow or discharge
	rhin/o = nose	**-scopy** = visual examination

1.86. A medical specialist concerned with the diagnosis and treatment of heart disease is a/an
_____.

1.87. The term meaning a runny nose is _____.

1.88. The term meaning the inflammation of a joint or joints is _____.

1.89. A medical specialist in disorders of the newborn is a/an _____.

1.90. The term meaning a surgical incision into a nerve is a/an _____.

1.91. The term meaning inflammation of the heart is _____.

1.92. The term meaning pain in the nose is _____.

1.93. The term meaning pain in a nerve or nerves is _____.

1.94. The term meaning a surgical incision into the heart is a/an _____.

1.95. The term meaning an inflammation of the nose is _____.

Labeling Exercises

1.96. The combining form meaning spinal cord is _____.

1.97. The combining form meaning muscle is _____.

1.98. The combining form meaning bone is _____.

1.99. The combining form meaning nerve is _____.

1.100. The combining form meaning joint is _____.

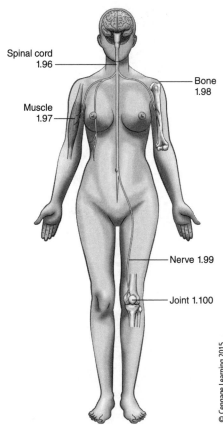

Spinal cord 1.96

Bone 1.98

Muscle 1.97

Nerve 1.99

Joint 1.100

© Cengage Learning 2015

The Human Body in Health and Disease

Learning Exercises

Class _____   Name _____

Matching Word Parts 1

Write the correct answer in the middle column.

Definition	Correct Answer	Possible Answers
2.1. fat	_____	**aden/o**
2.2. front	_____	**adip/o**
2.3. gland	_____	**anter/o**
2.4. specialist	_____	**-ologist**
2.5. study of	_____	**-ology**

Matching Word Parts 2

Write the correct answer in the middle column.

Definition	Correct Answer	Possible Answers
2.6. cell	_____	**caud/o**
2.7. head	_____	**cephal/o**
2.8. lower part of the body	_____	**cyt/o**
2.9. out of	_____	**endo-**
2.10. within	_____	**exo-**

Matching Word Parts 3

Write the correct answer in the middle column.

Definition	Correct Answer	Possible Answers
2.11. back	_____	**hist/o**
2.12. control	_____	**path/o**
2.13. disease, suffering, emotion	_____	**-plasia**
2.14. formation	_____	**poster/o**
2.15. tissue	_____	**-stasis**

Definitions

Select the correct answer, and write it on the line provided.

2.16. A/An _____ is acquired in a hospital setting.

    iatrogenic illness   idiopathic disorder   nosocomial infection   organic disorder

2.17. When a _____ is inherited from only one parent, the offspring will have that genetic condition or characteristic.

    dominant gene   genome   recessive gene   recessive trait

2.18. The _____ contains the major organs of digestion.

    abdominal cavity   cranial cavity   dorsal cavity   pelvic cavity

2.19. The term _____ means the direction toward or nearer the midline.

    distal   lateral   medial   proximal

2.20. The primary role of the undifferentiated _____ cells is to maintain and repair the tissue in which they are found.

    adult stem   cord blood   embryonic stem   hemopoietic

2.21. The genetic disorder in which an essential digestive enzyme is missing is known as _____.

    Down syndrome   Huntington's disease   phenylketonuria   Tay-Sachs disease

2.22. The inflammation of a gland is known as _____.

    adenectomy   adenitis   adenoma   adenosis

2.23. The _____ is the outer layer of the peritoneum that lines the interior of the abdominal wall.

    mesentery   parietal peritoneum   retroperitoneum   visceral peritoneum

2.24. A _____ is a fundamental physical and functional unit of heredity.

    cell   gamete   gene   genome

2.25. The study of the structure, composition, and function of tissues is known as _____.

    anatomy   cytology   histology   physiology

Matching Regions of the Thorax and Abdomen

Write the correct answer in the middle column.

Definition		Correct Answer	Possible Answers
2.26.	above the stomach	_____	epigastric region
2.27.	belly button area	_____	hypochondriac region
2.28.	below the ribs	_____	hypogastric region
2.29.	below the stomach	_____	iliac region
2.30.	hip bone area	_____	umbilical region

Which Word?

Select the correct answer, and write it on the line provided.

2.31. The term _____ refers to the entire lower area of the abdomen.

     inguinal   umbilicus

2.32. The study of how genes are transferred from parents to their children and the role of genes in health and disease is known as _____.

     cytology   genetics

2.33. A specialist in the study of the outbreaks of disease is a/an _____.

     epidemiologist   pathologist

2.34. The _____ secrete chemical substances into ducts.

     endocrine glands   exocrine glands

2.35. The location of the stomach is _____ to the diaphragm.

     inferior   superior

Spelling Counts

Find the misspelled word in each sentence. Then write that word, spelled correctly, on the line provided.

2.36. The mesantry is a fused double layer of the parietal peritoneum. _____

2.37. Hemaphilia is a group of hereditary bleeding disorders in which a blood-clotting factor is missing. _____

2.38. Hypretrophy is a general increase in the bulk of a body part or organ due to an increase in the size, but not in the number, of cells in the tissues. _____

2.39. The protective covering for all of the internal and external surfaces of the body is formed by epithealial tissues. _____

2.40. An abnomolly is any deviation from what is regarded as normal. _____

Abbreviation Identification

Write the correct terms for the abbreviations on the lines provided.

2.41. **HD** _____

2.42. **CD** _____

2.43. **GP** _____

2.44. **LUQ** _____

2.45. **CH** _____

Term Selection

Select the correct answer, and write it on the line provided.

2.46. The term meaning situated nearest the midline or beginning of a body structure is _____.

    distal   lateral   medial   proximal

2.47. The term meaning situated in the back is _____.

    anterior   posterior   superior   ventral

2.48. The body is divided into anterior and posterior portions by the _____ plane.

    frontal   horizontal   sagittal   transverse

2.49. The body is divided into equal vertical left and right halves by the _____ plane.

    coronal   midsagittal   sagittal   transverse

2.50. Part of the elbow is formed by the _____ end of the humerus.

    distal   lateral   medial   proximal

Sentence Completion

Write the correct term or terms on the lines provided.

2.51. _____ is a genetic variation that is associated with characteristic facial appearance, learning disabilities, and physical abnormalities such as heart valve disease.

2.52. The study of the functions of the structures of the body is known as _____.

2.53. The heart and the lungs are surrounded and protected by the _____ cavity.

2.54. An unfavorable response to prescribed medical treatment, such as severe burns resulting from radiation therapy, is known as a/an _____ illness.

2.55. The genetic structures located within the nucleus of each cell are known as _____. These structures are made up of the DNA molecules containing the body's genes.

Word Surgery

Divide each term into its component word parts. Write these word parts, in sequence, on the lines provided. When necessary use a slash (/) to indicate a combining vowel. (You may not need all of the lines provided.)

2.56. An **adenectomy** is the surgical removal of a gland.

_____ _____ _____ _____

2.57. Hormones are secreted directly into the bloodstream by the **endocrine** glands.

_____ _____ _____ _____

2.58. A **histologist** is a specialist in the study of the organization of tissues at all levels.

_____ _____ _____ _____

2.59. The term **retroperitoneal** means located behind the peritoneum.

_____ _____ _____ _____

2.60. A **pathologist** specializes in the laboratory analysis of tissue samples to confirm or establish a diagnosis.

_____ _____ _____ _____

2.61. The study of the causes of diseases is known as **etiology**.

_____ _____ _____ _____

2.62. The term **homeostasis** refers to the processes through which the body maintains a constant internal environment.

_____ _____ _____ _____

2.63. A **pandemic** is an outbreak of a disease occurring over a large geographic area, possibly worldwide.

_____ _____ _____ _____

2.64. The **epigastric** region is located above the stomach.

_____ _____ _____ _____

2.65. An **idiopathic** disorder is an illness without known cause.

_____ _____ _____ _____

Clinical Conditions

Write the correct answer on the line provided.

2.66. Mr. Tseng died of cholera during a sudden and widespread outbreak of this disease in his village. Such an outbreak is described as being a/an _____.

2.67. Brenda Farmer's doctor could not find any physical changes to explain her symptoms. The doctor refers to this as a/an _____ disorder.

2.68. Gerald Carlson was infected with hepatitis B through _____ transmission.

2.69. To become a specialist in the study and analysis of cells, Lee Wong signed up for courses in _____.

2.70. Malaria and West Nile virus are spread by mosquitoes. This is known as _____ transmission.

2.71. Jose Ortega complained of pain in the lower right area of his abdomen. Using the system that divides the abdomen into four sections, his doctor recorded the pain as being in the lower right _____.

2.72. Ralph Jenkins was very sick after drinking contaminated water during a camping trip. His doctor says that he contracted the illness through _____ transmission.

2.73. Tracy Ames has a bladder inflammation. This organ of the urinary system is located in the _____ cavity.

2.74. Mrs. Reynolds was diagnosed as having inflammation of the peritoneum. The medical term for this condition is _____.

2.75. Ashley Goldberg is fascinated by genetics. She wants to specialize in this field and is studying to become a/an _____.

Which Is the Correct Medical Term?

Select the correct answer, and write it on the line provided.

2.76. Debbie Sanchez fell against a rock and injured her left hip and upper leg. This area is known as the left _____ region.

hypochondriac   iliac   lumbar   umbilical

2.77. A _____ is the complete set of genetic information of an organism.

cell   gamete   gene   genome

2.78. An _____ is a malignant tumor that originates in glandular tissue.

adenocarcinoma   adenitis   adenoma   adenosis

2.79. Nerve cells and blood vessels are surrounded and supported by _____ connective tissue.

adipose   epithelial   liquid   loose

2.80. A mother's consumption of alcohol during pregnancy can cause _____.

cerebral palsy   Down syndrome   fetal alcohol syndrome   genetic disorders

Challenge Word Building

These terms are *not* found in this chapter; however, they are made up of the following familiar word parts. If you need help in creating the term, refer to your medical dictionary.

-algia	gastr/o	-itis
-ectomy	laryng/o	-osis
	neur/o	-plasty
	my/o	
	nephr/o	

2.81. The term meaning the surgical repair of a muscle is _____.

2.82. The term meaning muscle pain is _____.

2.83. The term meaning an abnormal condition of the stomach is _____.

2.84. The term meaning inflammation of the larynx is _____.

2.85. The term meaning the surgical removal of part of a muscle is a/an _____.

2.86. The term meaning pain in the stomach is _____.

2.87. The term meaning surgical removal of the larynx is _____.

2.88. The term meaning an abnormal condition of the kidney is _____.

2.89. The medical term meaning surgical repair of a nerve is _____.

2.90. The term meaning inflammation of the kidney is _____.

Labeling Exercises

Identify the numbered items in the accompanying figures.

2.91. This is the right _____ region.

2.92. This is the _____ region.

2.93. This is the _____ region.

2.94. This is the left _____ region.

2.95. This is the left _____ region.

2.96. This is the _____ plane, which is also known as the midline.

2.97. This is the _____ surface, which is also known as the ventral surface.

2.98. This arrow is pointing in a/an _____ direction.

2.99. This is the _____ surface, which is also known as the dorsal surface.

2.100. This is the _____ plane, which is a horizontal plane.

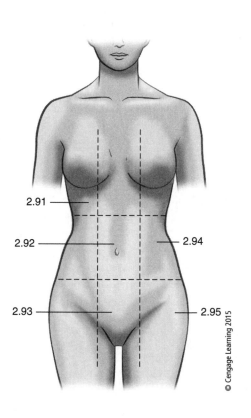

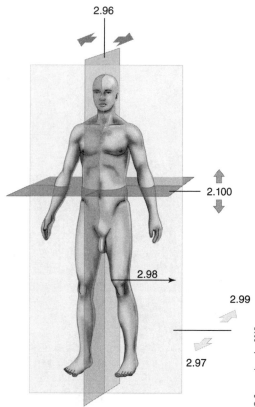

WORD PART REVIEW

The first two chapters of your textbook have introduced you to many word parts. In the next 13 chapters, you will learn about the body systems. You will find that mastering this information is much easier if you have already learned *at least some* of the word parts you met in the first two chapters.

This special **Word Part Review** is designed to reinforce your knowledge of these word parts and to confirm your mastery of them. To assist you with learning these word parts, this section is divided into two parts:

- The first part is **Word Part Practice.** It consists of 50 questions to provide practice in the use of the word parts you were introduced to in Chapters 1 and 2. It also provides opportunities to work with the use of combining vowels and word parts. If you are not certain of an answer, look it up in your textbook.

- The second part is a **Post-Test.** It includes 50 questions designed to enable you to evaluate your mastery of these word parts. Try to answer these questions without looking up the answers in Chapters 1 and 2.

If you are having problems in this section, ask your instructor for help NOW!

WORD PART PRACTICE SESSION

This is a practice session and you can go back into Chapters 1 and 2 to find the answers. This is a good idea because it gives you more experience in working with the terms and word parts found in these chapters.

Matching Word Roots and Their Meanings

Enter the correct **word root** in the middle column.

Definition	Correct Answer	Possible Answer
WP.1. joint	_____	**melan**
WP.2. skull	_____	**gastr**
WP.3. red	_____	**erythr**
WP.4. stomach	_____	**crani**
WP.5. black	_____	**arthr**

Matching Combining Forms and Their Meanings

Enter the correct **combining forms** in the middle column.

Definition		Correct Answer	Possible Answer
WP.6.	nose	_____	**aden/o**
WP.7.	liver	_____	**cardi/o**
WP.8.	gland	_____	**hepat/o**
WP.9.	heart	_____	**ot/o**
WP.10.	ear	_____	**rhin/o**

Matching Prefixes and Their Meanings

Enter the correct **prefix** in the middle column.

Definition		Correct Answer	Prefix
WP.11.	bad, difficult	_____	**intra-**
WP.12.	between, among	_____	**hypo-**
WP.13.	excessive, increased	_____	**hyper-**
WP.14.	within, inside	_____	**inter-**
WP.15.	deficient, decreased	_____	**dys-**

Matching Suffixes and Their Meanings

Enter the correct **suffix** in the middle column.

Definition		Correct Answer	Suffix
WP.16.	abnormal condition	_____	**-megaly**
WP.17.	bleeding	_____	**-ologist**
WP.18.	enlargement	_____	**-osis**
WP.19.	surgical repair	_____	**-plasty**
WP.20.	specialist	_____	**-rrhagia**

Matching Suffixes and Their Meanings

Enter the correct **suffix** in the middle column.

Definition		Correct Answer	Word Part
WP.21.	inflammation	_____	**-algia**
WP.22.	pain, suffering	_____	**-centesis**
WP.23.	process of producing a picture or record	_____	**-ectomy**
WP.24.	surgical puncture to remove fluid	_____	**-itis**
WP.25.	surgical removal	_____	**-graphy**

Matching Suffixes and Their Meanings

Enter the correct **suffix** in the middle column.

Definition	Correct Answer	Suffix
WP.26. abnormal flow, discharge	_____	**-oma**
WP.27. abnormal narrowing	_____	**-rrhaphy**
WP.28. tumor	_____	**-rrhea**
WP.29. rupture	_____	**-rrhexis**
WP.30. to suture	_____	**-stenosis**

Word Building

Write the word you create on the line provided.

WP.31. The term _____ means the surgical repair of the nose (**rhin/o** means nose).

WP.32. The term _____ means the surgical removal of a kidney (**nephr/o** means kidney).

WP.33. The term _____ means inflammation of the ear (**ot/o** means ear).

WP.34. The term _____ means the study of disorders of the blood (**hemat/o** means blood).

WP.35. The term _____ means inflammation of the liver (**hepat/o** means liver).

WP.36. The term _____ means the visual examination of the interior of a joint (**arthr/o** means joint).

WP.37. The term _____ means an inflammation of the appendix (**appendic** means appendix).

WP.38. The term _____ means a surgical incision into the colon (**col/o** means colon).

WP.39. The term _____ means the study of the functions of the structures of the body (**physi** means nature or physical).

WP.40. The term _____ (ECG) means a record or picture of the electrical activity of the heart (**electr/o** means electric, and **cardi/o** means heart).

True/False

If the word part definition is accurate, write **True** on the line. If the definition is not accurate, write **False** on the line.

WP.41. _____ **myc/o** means mucous.

WP.42. _____ **peri-** means surrounding.

WP.43. _____ **hypo-** means increased.

WP.44. _____ **ather/o** means plaque or fatty substance.

WP.45. _____ **-graphy** means the process of producing a picture or record.

WP.46. _____ **pyel/o** means pus.

WP.47. _____ **-ostomy** means the surgical creation of an artificial opening to the body surface.

WP.48. _____ **hist** means tissue.

WP.49. _____ **-centesis** means to see or a visual examination.

WP.50. _____ **-cyte** means cell.

WORD PART POST-TEST

Answer these questions without looking them up in Chapters 1 and 2. If you have trouble, you should arrange to get extra help or practice more in working with word parts.

Write the word part on the line provided.

PT.1.   The **suffix** meaning surgical removal is _____.

PT.2.   The **prefix** meaning under, less, or below is _____.

PT.3.   The **suffix** meaning surgical repair is _____.

PT.4.   The **combining form** meaning fungus is _____.

PT.5.   The **combining form** meaning joint is _____.

PT.6.   The **combining form** meaning muscle is _____.

PT.7.   The **prefix** meaning between or among is _____.

PT.8.   The **combining form** meaning bone marrow or spinal cord is _____.

PT.9.   The **suffix** meaning a visual examination is _____.

PT.10. The **suffix** meaning the study of is _____.

Matching Word Parts 1

Matching Suffixes and Prefixes with Their Meanings

Enter the correct **word part** in the middle column.

Definition	Correct Answer	Possible Answer
PT.11. tumor	_____	**arteri/o**
PT.12. surgical suturing	_____	**-oma**
PT.13. surrounding	_____	**peri-**
PT.14. rupture	_____	**-rrhaphy**
PT.15. artery	_____	**-rrhexis**

Matching Word Parts 2

Matching Suffixes and Prefixes with Their Meanings

Enter the correct **word part** in the middle column.

Definition	Correct Answer	Possible Answer
PT.16. abnormal hardening	_____	**dys-**
PT.17. bad, difficult, painful	_____	**-itis**
PT.18. inflammation	_____	**-ostomy**
PT.19. surgical creation of an artificial opening	_____	**-osis**
PT.20. abnormal condition or disease	_____	**-sclerosis**

True/False

If the statement is accurate, write **True** on the line. If the statement is not correct, write **False** on the line.

PT.21. _____ The combining form **hem/o** means blood.

PT.22. _____ The suffix **-algia** means pain.

PT.23. _____ The combining form **oste/o** means bone.

PT.24. _____ The prefix **hyper-** means deficient or decreased.

PT.25. _____ The combining form **rhin/o** means nose.

Word Surgery

Use your knowledge of word parts to identify the parts of these terms. Write the word parts, in sequence, on the lines provided. When necessary, use a slash (/) to indicate a combining vowel.

PT.26. The term meaning the surgical repair of a nerve is **neuroplasty**. This word is made up of the word parts _____ and _____.

PT.27. The term describing any pathological change or disease in the spinal cord is **myelopathy**. This term is made up of the word parts _____ and _____.

PT.28. The medical condition **pyrosis** is commonly known as heartburn. This term is made up of the word parts _____ and _____.

PT.29. The **endocrine** glands produce hormones, but do not have ducts. This term is made up of the word parts _____ and _____.

PT.30. The term meaning a mature red blood cell is **erythrocyte**. This term is made up of the word parts _____ and _____.

Word Building

Write the word you created on the line provided.

Regarding Nerves (neur/o means nerve)

PT.31. A surgical incision into a nerve is a/an _____.

PT.32. The study of the nervous system is known as _____.

PT.33. The surgical repair of a nerve or nerves is a/an _____.

PT.34. The term meaning to suture the ends of a severed nerve is _____.

PT.35. Abnormal softening of the nerves is called _____.

PT.36. A specialist in diagnosing and treating disorders of the nervous system is a/an _____.

PT.37. The term meaning inflammation of a nerve or nerves is _____.

Relating to Blood Vessels (angi/o means relating to the blood vessels)

PT.38. The death of the walls of blood vessels is _____.

PT.39. The abnormal hardening of the walls of blood vessels is _____.

PT.40. The abnormal narrowing of a blood vessel is _____.

PT.41. The surgical removal of a blood vessel is a/an _____.

PT.42. The process of recording a picture of blood vessels is called _____.

Missing Words

Write the missing word on the line provided.

PT.43. The surgical repair of an artery is a/an _____ (**arteri/o** means artery).

PT.44. The medical term meaning inflammation of the larynx is _____ (**laryng/o** means larynx).

PT.45. The surgical removal of all or part of the colon is a/an _____ (**col/o** means colon).

PT.46. The abnormal softening of muscle tissue is _____ (**my/o** means muscle).

PT.47. The term meaning any abnormal condition of the stomach is _____ (**gastr/o** means stomach).

PT.48. The term meaning the study of the heart is _____ (**cardi/o** means heart).

PT.49. The term meaning inflammation of the colon is _____ (**col/o** means colon).

PT.50. The term meaning a surgical incision into a vein is _____ (**phleb/o** means vein).

CHAPTER 3

The Skeletal System

Learning Exercises

Class _____   Name _____

Matching Word Parts 1

Write the correct answer in the middle column.

Definition	Correct Answer	Possible Answers
3.1. hump	_____	**ankyl/o**
3.2. cartilage	_____	**arthr/o**
3.3. crooked, bent, stiff	_____	**-um**
3.4. joint	_____	**kyph/o**
3.5. singular noun ending	_____	**chondr/i, chondr/o**

Matching Word Parts 2

Write the correct answer in the middle column.

Definition	Correct Answer	Possible Answers
3.6. cranium, skull	_____	**cost/o**
3.7. rib	_____	**crani/o**
3.8. setting free, loosening	_____	**-desis**
3.9. spinal cord, bone marrow	_____	**-lysis**
3.10. to bind, tie together	_____	**myel/o**

Matching Word Parts 3

Write the correct answer in the middle column.

Definition	Correct Answer	Possible Answers
3.11. vertebrae	_____	**oste/o**
3.12. curved	_____	**spondyl/o**
3.13. swayback bent	_____	**lord/o**
3.14. synovial membrane	_____	**synovi/o, synov/o**
3.15. bone	_____	**scoli/o**

Definitions

Select the correct answer, and write it on the line provided.

3.16. The shaft of a long bone is known as the _____.

diaphysis   distal epiphysis   endosteum   proximal epiphysis

3.17. Seven short _____ bones make up each ankle.

carpal   metatarsal   phalanx   tarsal

3.18. The upper portion of the sternum is the _____.

clavicle   mandible   manubrium   xiphoid process

3.19. A _____ is movable.

cartilaginous joint   fibrous joint   suture joint   synovial joint

3.20. The _____ bone is located just below the urinary bladder.

ilium   ischium   pubis   sacrum

3.21. The opening in a bone through which blood vessels, nerves, and ligaments pass is a _____.

foramen   foramina   process   symphysis

3.22. A/An _____ connects one bone to another bone.

articular cartilage   ligament   synovial membrane   phalange

3.23. The hip socket is known as the _____.

acetabulum   malleolus   patella   trochanter

3.24. The bones of the fingers and toes are known as the _____.

carpals   metatarsals   tarsals   phalanges

3.25. A normal projection on the surface of a bone that serves as an attachment for muscles and tendons is known as a/an _____.

cruciate   exostosis   popliteal   process

Matching Structures

Write the correct answer in the middle column.

Definition	Correct Answer	Possible Answers
3.26. breast bone	_____	clavicle
3.27. cheekbones	_____	olecranon process
3.28. collar bone	_____	sternum
3.29. kneecap	_____	patella
3.30. point of the elbow	_____	zygomatic

Which Word?

Select the correct answer, and write it on the line provided.

3.31. The surgical procedure for loosening of an ankylosed joint is known as _____.

    arthrodesis   arthrolysis

3.32. The bone disorder of unknown cause that destroys normal bone structure and replaces it with fibrous (scarlike) tissue is known as _____.

    fibrous dysplasia   Paget's disease

3.33. An _____ bone marrow transplant uses bone marrow from a donor.

    allogenic   autologous

3.34. A percutaneous _____ is performed to treat osteoporosis-related compression fractures.

    diskectomy   vertebroplasty

3.35. The medical term for the form of arthritis that is commonly known as wear-and-tear arthritis is _____.

    osteoarthritis   rheumatoid arthritis

Spelling Counts

Find the misspelled word in each sentence. Then write that word, spelled correctly, on the line provided.

3.36. The medical term for the condition commonly known as low back pain is lumbaego.

_____

3.37. The surgical fracture of a bone to correct a deformity is known as osteclasis.

_____

3.38. Ankylosing spondilitis is a form of rheumatoid arthritis that primarily causes inflammation of the joints between the vertebrae. _____

3.39. An osterrhaphy is the surgical suturing, or wiring together, of bones. _____

3.40. Crepetation is the grating sound heard when the ends of a broken bone move together.

_____

Abbreviation Identification

Write the correct answer on the line provided.

3.41. **BMT** _____

3.42. **CR** _____

3.43. **Fx** _____

3.44. **RA** _____

3.45. **TMJ** _____

Term Selection

Select the correct answer, and write it on the line provided.

3.46. The term meaning the death of bone tissue is _____.

    osteitis deformans   osteomyelitis   osteonecrosis   osteoporosis

3.47. An abnormal increase in the forward curvature of the lumbar spine is known as

    _____.

    kyphosis   lordosis   scoliosis   spondylosis

3.48. The condition known as _____ is a congenital defect.

    juvenile arthritis   osteoarthritis   rheumatoid arthritis   spina bifida

3.49. A type of cancer that occurs in blood-making cells found in the red bone marrow is known as a/an

    _____.

    chondroma   Ewing's sarcoma   myeloma   osteochondroma

3.50. The bulging deposit that forms around the area of the break during the healing of a fractured bone is a _____.

    callus   crepitation   crepitus   luxation

Sentence Completion

Write the correct term or terms on the lines provided.

3.51. A/An _____ is performed to gain access to the brain or to relieve intracranial pressure.

3.52. The partial displacement of a bone from its joint is known as _____.

3.53. The procedure that stiffens a joint by joining two bones is _____. This is also known as surgical ankylosis.

3.54. The surgical placement of an artificial joint is known as _____.

3.55. A medical term for the condition commonly known as a bunion is _____.

Word Surgery

Divide each term into its component word parts. Write these word parts, in sequence, on the lines provided. When necessary, use a slash (/) to indicate a combining vowel. (You may not need all of the lines provided.)

3.56. **Hemarthrosis** is blood within a joint.

_____   _____   _____   _____

3.57. An **osteochondroma** is a benign bony projection covered with cartilage.

_____   _____   _____   _____

3.58. **Osteomalacia**, also known as adult rickets, is abnormal softening of bones in adults.

_____   _____   _____   _____

3.59. **Periostitis** is an inflammation of the periosteum.

_____   _____   _____   _____

3.60. **Spondylolisthesis** is the forward slipping movement of the body of one of the lower lumbar vertebrae on the vertebra or sacrum below it.

_____   _____   _____   _____

True/False

If the statement is true, write **True** on the line. If the statement is false, write **False** on the line.

3.61. _____ Osteopenia is thinner-than-average bone density. This term is used to describe the condition of someone who does not yet have osteoporosis, but is at risk for developing it.

3.62. _____ Paget's disease is caused by a deficiency of calcium and vitamin D in early childhood.

3.63. _____ Costochondritis is an inflammation of the cartilage that connects a rib to the sternum.

3.64. _____ Dislocation is the partial displacement of a bone from its joint.

3.65. _____ Arthroscopic surgery is a minimally invasive procedure for the treatment of the interior of a joint.

Clinical Conditions

Write the correct answer on the line provided.

3.66. When Bobby Kuhn fell out of a tree, the bone in his arm was bent and partially broken. Dr. Grafton described this as a/an _____ fracture and told the family that this type of fracture occurs primarily in children.

3.67. Eduardo Sanchez was treated for an inflammation of the bone and bone marrow. The medical term for this condition is _____.

3.68. Beth Hubert's breast cancer spread to her bones. These new sites are referred to as

_____.

3.69. Mrs. Morton suffers from dowager's hump. The medical term for this abnormal curvature of the spine is _____.

3.70. Henry Turner wears a brace to compensate for the impaired function of his leg. The medical term for this orthopedic appliance is a/an _____.

3.71. As the result of a head injury in an auto accident, Sam Cheng required a/an _____ to relieve the rapidly increasing intracranial pressure.

3.72. Mrs. Gilmer has leukemia and requires a bone marrow transplant. Part of the treatment was the harvesting of her bone marrow so she could receive it later as a/an _____ bone marrow transplant.

3.73. Betty Greene has been running for several years; however, now her knees hurt. Dr. Morita diagnosed her condition as _____, which is an abnormal softening of the cartilage in these joints.

3.74. Patty Turner (age 7) has symptoms that include a skin rash, fever, slowed growth, fatigue, and swelling in the joints. She was diagnosed as having juvenile _____ arthritis.

3.75. Heather Lewis has a very sore shoulder. Dr. Plunkett diagnosed this as an inflammation of the bursa and said that Heather's condition is _____.

Which Is the Correct Medical Term?

Select the correct answer, and write it on the line provided.

3.76. Rodney Horner is being treated for a _____ fracture in which the ends of the bones were crushed together.

    Colles'   comminuted   compound   spiral

3.77. Alex Jordon fell and injured her knee. Her doctor performed a/an _____ to surgically repair the damaged cartilage.

    arthroplasty   chondroma   chondroplasty   osteoplasty

3.78. Mrs. Palmer is at high risk for osteoporosis. To obtain a definitive evaluation of the status of her bone density, Mrs. Palmer's physician ordered a/an _____ test.

    dual x-ray absorptiometry   MRI   x-ray   ultrasonic bone density

3.79. In an effort to return a fractured bone to normal alignment, Dr. Wong ordered _____. This procedure exerts a pulling force on the distal end of the affected limb.

    external fixation   immobilization   internal fixation   traction

3.80. Baby Juanita was treated for _____, which is a congenital deformity of the foot involving the talus (ankle bones). Her family calls this condition clubfoot.

    osteomalacia   rickets   scoliosis   talipes

Challenge Word Building

These terms are *not* found in this chapter; however, they are made up of the following familiar word parts. If you need help in creating the term, refer to your medical dictionary.

poly-	**arthr/o**	**-ectomy**
	chondr/o	**-itis**
	cost/o	**-malacia**
	crani/o	**-otomy**
	oste/o	**-pathy**
		-sclerosis

3.81. Abnormal hardening of bone is known as _____.

3.82. The surgical removal of a rib or ribs is a/an _____.

3.83. Any disease of cartilage is known as _____.

3.84. A surgical incision into a joint is a/an _____.

3.85. Inflammation of cartilage is known as _____.

3.86. The surgical removal of a joint is a/an _____.

3.87. Inflammation of more than one joint is known as _____.

3.88. Any disease involving the bones and joints is known as _____.

3.89. A surgical incision or division of a rib or ribs is a/an _____.

3.90. Abnormal softening of the skull is known as _____.

Labeling Exercises

Identify the numbered items on the accompanying figures.

3.91. _____ vertebrae

3.92. _____

3.93. _____

3.94. _____

3.95. _____

3.96. _____

3.97. _____ bone

3.98. _____ bone

3.99. _____ bone

3.100. _____

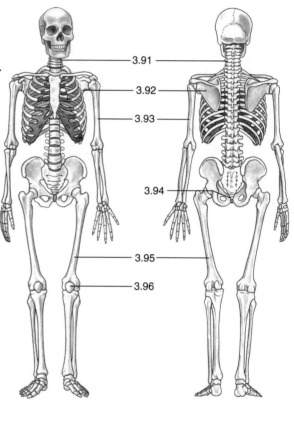

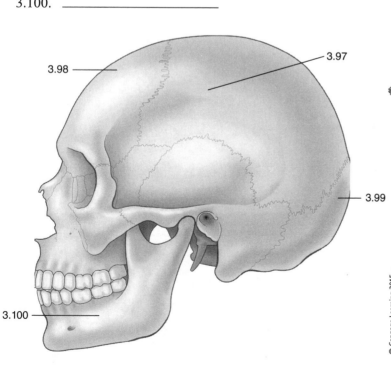

The Muscular System

Learning Exercises

Class _____   Name _____

Matching Word Parts 1

Write the correct answer in the middle column.

Definition	Correct Answer	Possible Answers
4.1. abnormal condition	_____	-cele
4.2. fascia	_____	fasci/o
4.3. fibrous tissue	_____	fibr/o
4.4. hernia, swelling	_____	-ia
4.5. movement	_____	kines/o, kinesi/o

Matching Word Parts 2

Write the correct answer in the middle column.

Definition	Correct Answer	Possible Answers
4.6. coordination	_____	my/o
4.7. muscle	_____	-rrhexis
4.8. rupture	_____	tax/o
4.9. tendon	_____	tend/o
4.10. tone	_____	ton/o

Matching Muscle Directions and Positions

Write the correct answer in the middle column.

Definition	Correct Answer	Possible Answers
4.11. crosswise	_____	lateralis
4.12. ringlike	_____	oblique
4.13. slanted at an angle	_____	rectus
4.14. straight	_____	sphincter
4.15. toward the side	_____	transverse

Definitions

Select the correct answer, and write it on the line provided.

4.16. The _____ muscles are under voluntary control.

    involuntary   nonstriated   skeletal   visceral

4.17. A/An _____ is a calcium deposit in the plantar fascia near its attachment to the calcaneus bone.

    heel spur   impingement syndrome   overuse injury   shin splint

4.18. Turning the hand so the palm is upward is called _____.

    extension   flexion   pronation   supination

4.19. One of the symptoms of Parkinson's disease is _____, which is extreme slowness of movement.

    bradykinesia   dyskinesia   hypotonia   hyperactivity

4.20. A/An _____ is a physician who specializes in physical medicine and rehabilitation with the focus on restoring function.

    exercise physiologist   physiatrist   physiologist   rheumatologist

4.21. The term _____ means pertaining to muscle tissue and fascia.

    aponeurosis   fibrous sheath   myocardium   myofascial

4.22. A/An _____ is a narrow band of nonelastic, fibrous connective tissue that attaches a muscle to a bone.

    aponeurosis   fascia   ligament   tendon

4.23. A band of fibers that holds structures together abnormally is a/an _____. These bands can form as the result of an injury or surgery.

    adhesion   aponeurosis   atrophy   contracture

4.24. The paralysis of both legs and the lower part of the body is known as _____.

    hemiparesis   hemiplegia   paraplegia   quadriplegia

4.25. The surgical suturing of the end of a tendon to a bone is known as _____.

    tenodesis   tenorrhaphy   tendinosis   tenolysis

Matching Structures

Write the correct answer in the middle column.

Definition	Correct Answer	Possible Answers
4.26. heart muscle	_____	gluteus maximus
4.27. buttock muscle	_____	myocardial
4.28. fibrous connective tissue	_____	sphincter
4.29. muscular cap of shoulder	_____	tendon
4.30. ring-like muscle	_____	deltoid

Which Word?

Select the correct answer, and write it on the line provided.

4.31. An injury to the body of the muscle or the attachment of a tendon is known as a/an _____. These are usually associated with overuse injuries that involve a wrenched or torn muscle or tendon attachment.

    sprain   strain

4.32. A _____ is a drug that causes temporary paralysis by blocking the transmission of nerve stimuli to the muscles.

    neuromuscular blocker   skeletal muscle relaxant

4.33. The condition of abnormal muscle tone that causes the impairment of voluntary muscle movement is known as _____.

    ataxia   dystonia

4.34. Inflamed and swollen tendons caught in the narrow space between the bones within the shoulder joint cause the condition known as _____.

    impingement syndrome   intermittent claudication

4.35. The _____ forms the muscular cap of the shoulder.

    triceps brachii   deltoid

Spelling Counts

Find the misspelled word in each sentence. Then write that word, spelled correctly, on the line provided.

4.36. An antispasmydic is administered to suppress smooth muscle contractions of the stomach, intestine, or bladder. _____

4.37. The medical term for hiccups is singulutas. _____

4.38. Myasthenia gravus is a chronic autoimmune disease that affects the neuromuscular junction and produces serious weakness of voluntary muscles. _____

4.39. A ganglian cyst is a harmless fluid-filled swelling that occurs most commonly on the outer surface of the wrist. _____

4.40. Pronetion is the movement that turns the palm of the hand downward or backward. _____

Abbreviation Identification

Write the correct answer on the line provided.

4.41. **CTS** _____

4.42. **DTR** _____

4.43. **ROM** _____

4.44. **RSD** _____

4.45. **SCI** _____

Term Selection

Select the correct answer, and write it on the line provided.

4.46. The term _____ means the rupture or tearing of a muscle.

   myocele   myorrhaphy   myorrhexis   myotomy

4.47. The term meaning the degeneration of muscle tissue is _____.

   myoclonus   myolysis   myocele   myoparesis

4.48. The term _____ means abnormally increased muscle function or activity.

   hyperkinesia   hypertonia   dyskinesia   hypotonia

4.49. A/An _____ injury can be a strain or tear on any of the three muscles that straighten the hip and bend the knee.

   Achilles tendon   hamstring   myofascial   shin splint

4.50. The specialized soft-tissue manipulation technique used to ease the pain of conditions such as fibromyalgia syndrome, movement restrictions, and temporomandibular joint disorders is known as _____.

   myofascial release   occupational therapy   RICE   therapeutic ultrasound

Sentence Completion

Write the correct term or terms on the lines provided.

4.51. An inflammation of the tissues surrounding the elbow is known as _____.

4.52. The movement during which the knees or elbows are bent to decrease the angle of the joints is known as _____.

4.53. Pain in the leg muscles that occurs during exercise and is relieved by rest is known as _____. This condition is due to poor circulation and is associated with peripheral vascular disease.

4.54. A weakness or slight muscular paralysis is known as _____.

4.55. A stiff neck due to spasmodic contraction of the neck muscles that pull the head toward the affected side is known as _____ or wryneck.

Word Surgery

Divide each term into its component word parts. Write these word parts, in sequence, on the lines provided. When necessary, use a slash (/) to indicate a combining vowel. (You may not need all of the lines provided.)

4.56. **Electromyography** is a diagnostic test that measures the electrical activity within muscle fibers.

_____   _____   _____   _____

4.57. **Hyperkinesia** means abnormally increased muscle function or activity.

_____   _____   _____   _____

4.58. **Myoclonus** is the sudden, involuntary jerking of a muscle or group of muscles.

_____   _____   _____   _____

4.59. **Polymyositis** is a muscle disease characterized by the simultaneous inflammation and weakening of voluntary muscles in many parts of the body.

_____   _____   _____   _____

4.60. **Sarcopenia** is the loss of muscle mass, strength, and function that comes with aging.

_____   _____   _____   _____

True/False

If the statement is true, write **True** on the line. If the statement is false, write **False** on the line.

4.61. _____ Overuse tendinitis is inflammation of tendons caused by excessive or unusual use of a joint.

4.62. _____ Hemiplegia is the total paralysis of the lower half of the body.

4.63. _____ A spasm is a sudden, involuntary contraction of one or more muscles.

4.64. _____ Ataxia is the distortion of voluntary movement such as in a tic or spasm.

4.65. _____ Striated muscles are located in the walls of internal organs such as the digestive tract, blood vessels, and ducts leading from glands.

Clinical Conditions

Write the correct answer on the line provided.

4.66. George Quinton developed a swelling on the outer surface of his wrist. His doctor diagnosed this as being a/an _____ and explained that this was a harmless fluid-filled swelling.

4.67. Raul Valladares has a protrusion of a muscle substance through a tear in the fascia surrounding it. This condition is known as a/an _____.

4.68. Louisa Ferraro experienced _____ of her leg muscles due to the disuse of these muscles over a long period of time.

4.69. Jasmine Franklin has _____. This is a condition in which there is diminished tone of the skeletal muscles.

4.70. Carolyn Goodwin complained of profound fatigue that is not improved by bed rest and was made worse by physical or mental activity. After ruling out other causes, her physician diagnosed her condition as being _____ syndrome.

4.71. Chuan Lee, who is a runner, required treatment for _____. This condition is a painful inflammation of the Achilles tendon caused by excessive stress being placed on that tendon.

4.72. For the first several days after his fall, Bob Hill suffered severe muscle pain. This condition is known as _____.

4.73. Jorge Guendulay could not play for his team because of a/an _____. This is a painful condition caused by the muscle tearing away from the tibia.

4.74. Due to a spinal cord injury, Marissa Giannati suffers from _____, which is paralysis of all four limbs.

4.75. Duncan McDougle has slight paralysis on one side of his body. This condition, which was caused by a stroke, is known as _____.

Which Is the Correct Medical Term?

Select the correct answer, and write it on the line provided.

4.76. The term *muscular* _____ describes a group of genetic diseases characterized by progressive weakness and degeneration of the skeletal muscles.

atonic   ataxia   dystonia   dystrophy

4.77. The surgical enlargement of the carpal tunnel or cutting of the carpal ligament to relieve nerve pressure is called _____.

carpal tunnel syndrome   compartment syndrome   carpal tunnel release   myofascial pain syndrome

4.78. During _____, the arm moves inward and toward the side of the body.

abduction   adduction   circumduction   rotation

4.79. A surgical incision into a muscle is known as _____.

myocele   myorrhaphy   myotomy   fascioplasty

4.80. The term _____ means bending the foot upward at the ankle.

abduction   dorsiflexion   elevation   plantar flexion

Challenge Word Building

These terms are *not* found in this chapter; however, they are made up of the following familiar word parts. If you need help in creating the term, refer to your medical dictionary.

poly-	card/o	-desis
	fasci/o	-ectomy
	herni/o	-itis
	my/o	-necrosis
	sphincter/o	-otomy
		-pathy
		-rrhaphy
		-algia

4.81. Any abnormal condition of skeletal muscles is known as _____.

4.82. Pain in several muscle groups is known as _____.

4.83. The death of individual muscle fibers is known as _____.

4.84. Surgical suturing of torn fascia is known as _____.

4.85. Based on word parts, the removal of multiple muscles is known as _____.

4.86. The surgical attachment of a fascia to another fascia or to a tendon is known as
_____.

4.87. Inflammation of the muscle of the heart is known as _____.

4.88. The surgical removal of fascia is a/an _____.

4.89. The surgical suturing of a defect in a muscular wall, such as the repair of a hernia, is a/an
_____.

4.90. An incision into a sphincter muscle is a/an _____.

Labeling Exercises

Identify the movements in the accompanying figures by writing the correct term on the line provided.

4.91. _____

4.92. _____

4.93. _____

4.94. _____

4.95. _____

4.96. _____

4.97. _____

4.98. _____

4.99. _____

4.100. _____

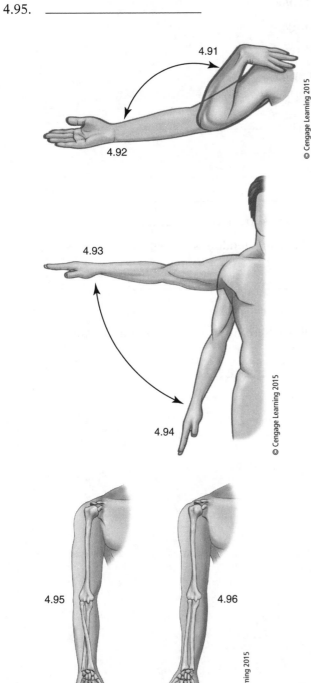

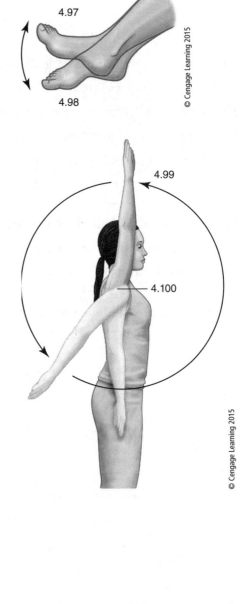

CHAPTER 5

The Cardiovascular System

Learning Exercises

Class _____   Name _____

Matching Word Parts 1

Write the correct answer in the middle column.

Definition	Correct Answer	Possible Answers
5.1. aorta	_____	**angi/o**
5.2. artery	_____	**aort/o**
5.3. plaque, fatty substance	_____	**arteri/o**
5.4. relating to blood or lymph vessels	_____	**ather/o**
5.5. slow	_____	**brady-**

Matching Word Parts 2

Write the correct answer in the middle column.

Definition	Correct Answer	Possible Answers
5.6. blood or blood condition	_____	**cardi/o**
5.7. heart	_____	**-crasia**
5.8. mixture or blending	_____	**ven/o**
5.9. red	_____	**-emia**
5.10. vein	_____	**erythr/o**

Matching Word Parts 3

Write the correct answer in the middle column.

Definition	Correct Answer	Possible Answers
5.11. white	_____	**hem/o**
5.12. vein	_____	**leuk/o**
5.13. fast, rapid	_____	**phleb/o**
5.14. clot	_____	**tachy-**
5.15. blood, relating to blood	_____	**thromb/o**

Definitions

Select the correct answer, and write it on the line provided.

5.16. The term meaning white blood cells is _____.

    erythrocytes   leukocytes   platelets   thrombocytes

5.17. Commonly known as the natural pacemaker, the medical name of the structure is the _____.

    atrioventricular node   bundle of His   Purkinje fiber   sinoatrial node

5.18. The myocardium receives its blood supply from the _____ arteries.

    aorta   coronary arteries   inferior vena cava   superior vena cava

5.19. The _____ are formed in red bone marrow and then migrate to tissues throughout the body. These blood cells destroy parasitic organisms and play a major role in allergic reactions.

    basophils   eosinophils   erythrocytes   monocytes

5.20. The bicuspid valve is also known as the _____ valve.

    aortic   mitral   pulmonary   tricuspid

5.21. The _____ pumps blood into the pulmonary artery, which carries it to the lungs.

    left atrium   left ventricle   right atrium   right ventricle

5.22. The _____ are the smallest formed elements in the blood, and they play an important role in blood clotting.

    erythrocytes   leukocytes   monocytes   thrombocytes

5.23. A foreign object, such as a bit of tissue or air, circulating in the blood is known as a/an _____.

    embolism   embolus   thrombosis   thrombus

5.24. The _____ carries blood to all parts of the body except the lungs.

    left atrium   left ventricle   right atrium   right ventricle

5.25. The _____ are the most common type of white blood cell.

    erythrocytes   leukocytes   neutrophils   thrombocytes

Matching Structures

Write the correct answer in the middle column.

Definition	Correct Answer	Possible Answers
5.26. a hollow, muscular organ	_____	endocardium
5.27. cardiac muscle	_____	epicardium
5.28. external layer of the heart	_____	heart
5.29. inner lining of the heart	_____	myocardium
5.30. sac enclosing the heart	_____	pericardium

Which Word?

Select the correct answer, and write it on the line provided.

5.31. High-density _____ is also known as good cholesterol.

   lipoprotein cholesterol   total cholesterol

5.32. An abnormally slow resting heart rate is described as _____.

   bradycardia   tachycardia

5.33. In _____ fibrillation, instead of pumping strongly, the heart muscle quivers ineffectively.

   atrial   ventricular

5.34. The highest pressure against the blood vessels is _____ pressure, and it occurs when the ventricles contract.

   diastolic   systolic

5.35. The diagnostic procedure that images the structures of the blood vessels and the flow of blood through these vessels is known as _____.

   digital angiography   duplex ultrasound

Spelling Counts

Find the misspelled word in each sentence. Then write that word, spelled correctly, on the line provided.

5.36. The autopsy indicated that the cause of death was a ruptured aneuryism. _____

5.37. A deficiency of blood passing through an organ or body part is known as hypoprefusion. _____

5.38. An arrhythemia is an abnormal heart rhythm in which the heartbeat is faster or slower than normal. _____

5.39. Reynaud's disease is a condition with symptoms that include intermittent attacks of pallor, cyanosis, and redness of the fingers and toes. _____

5.40. An automated implantable cardioverter-defibrilator is a double-action pacemaker. _____

Abbreviation Identification

In the space provided, write the words that each abbreviation stands for.

5.41. **CAD** _____

5.42. **EKG, ECG** _____

5.43. **A-fib** _____

5.44. **MI** _____

5.45. **V-fib** _____

Term Selection

Select the correct answer, and write it on the line provided.

5.46. The systemic condition often associated with severe infections caused by the presence of bacteria in the blood is known as _____.

    dyscrasia   endocarditis   pericarditis   septicemia

5.47. A/An _____ reduces the workload of the heart by slowing the rate of the heartbeat.

    ACE inhibitor   beta-blocker   calcium blocker   statin inhibitor

5.48. The blood disorder characterized by anemia in which the red blood cells are larger than normal is known as _____ anemia.

    aplastic   hemolytic   megaloblastic   pernicious

5.49. A/An _____ is a class of drugs administered to lower high blood pressure.

    antiarrhythmic   antihypertensive   aspirin   diuretic

5.50. A bacterial infection of the lining or valves of the heart is known as bacterial

_____.

    endocarditis   myocarditis   pericarditis   valvulitis

Sentence Completion

Write the correct term or terms on the lines provided.

5.51. Plasma with the clotting proteins removed is known as _____.

5.52. Having an abnormally small number of platelets in the circulating blood is known as

_____.

5.53. The surgical removal of the lining of a portion of a clogged carotid artery leading to the brain is known as a/an _____.

5.54. The abnormal protrusion of a heart valve that results in the inability of the valve to close completely is known as a/an _____.

5.55. The medication _____ is prescribed to prevent or relieve the pain of angina by dilating the blood vessels to the heart.

Word Surgery

Divide each term into its component word parts. Write these word parts, in sequence, on the lines provided. When necessary, use a slash (/) to indicate a combining vowel. (You may not need all of the lines provided.)

5.56. **Aneurysmorrhaphy** means the surgical suturing of a ruptured aneurysm.

_____ _____ _____ _____

5.57. **Aplastic** anemia is characterized by an absence of *all* formed blood elements.

_____ _____ _____ _____

5.58. **Electrocardiography** is the process of recording the electrical activity of the myocardium.

_____ _____ _____ _____

5.59. **Polyarteritis** is a form of vasculitis involving several medium and small arteries at the same time.

_____ _____ _____ _____

5.60. **Valvoplasty** is the surgical repair or replacement of a heart valve.

_____ _____ _____ _____

True/False

If the statement is true, write **True** on the line. If the statement is false, write **False** on the line.

5.61. _____ A thrombus is a clot or piece of tissue circulating in the blood.

5.62. _____ Hemochromatosis is also known as iron overload disease.

5.63. _____ Plasmapheresis is the removal of whole blood from the body, separation of its cellular elements, and reinfusion of these cellular elements suspended in saline or a plasma substitute.

5.64. _____ A vasoconstrictor is a drug that enlarges the blood vessels.

5.65. _____ Peripheral vascular disease is a disorder of the blood vessels located outside the heart and brain.

Clinical Conditions

Write the correct answer on the line provided.

5.66. Alberta Fleetwood has a/an _____. This condition is a benign tumor made up of newly formed blood vessels.

5.67. After his surgery, Ramon Martinez developed a deep vein _____ in his leg.

5.68. During her pregnancy, Polly Olson suffered from abnormally swollen veins in her legs. The medical term for this condition is _____ veins.

5.69. Thomas Wilkerson suffers from episodes of severe chest pain due to inadequate blood flow to the myocardium. This is a condition known as _____.

5.70. When Mr. Klein stands up too quickly, his blood pressure drops. His physician describes this as postural or _____ _____.

5.71. Juanita Gomez was diagnosed as having _____. This bone marrow disorder is characterized by the insufficient production of one or more types of blood cells.

5.72. Dr. Lawson read her patient's _____. This diagnostic record is also known as an ECG or EKG.

5.73. Jason Turner suffered from cardiac arrest. The paramedics arrived promptly and saved his life by using _____ (CPR).

5.74. Darlene Nolan was diagnosed as having a deep vein thrombosis. Her doctor immediately prescribed a/an _____ to cause the thrombus to dissolve.

5.75. Hamilton Edwards Sr. suffers from _____ (IHD). This is a group of cardiac disabilities resulting from an insufficient supply of oxygenated blood to the heart.

Which Is the Correct Medical Term?

Select the correct answer, and write it on the line provided.

5.76. A/An _____, which is a characteristic of atherosclerosis, is a deposit of plaque on or within the arterial wall.

vasculitis   angiostenosis   arteriosclerosis   atheroma

5.77. The term _____ means to stop or control bleeding.

hemochromatosis   hemostasis   plasmapheresis   transfusion reaction

5.78. Inflammation of a vein is known as _____.

arteriostenosis   endocarditis   phlebitis   carditis

5.79. Blood _____ is any pathologic condition of the cellular elements of the blood.

anemia   dyscrasia   hemochromatosis   septicemia

5.80. The surgical removal of an aneurysm is a/an _____.

aneurysmectomy   aneurysmoplasty   aneurysmorrhaphy   aneurysmotomy

Challenge Word Building

These terms are *not* found in this chapter; however, they are made up of the following familiar word parts. If you need help in creating the term, refer to your medical dictionary.

peri-	**angi/o**	**-itis**
	arter/o	**-necrosis**
	cardi/o	**-rrhaphy**
	phleb/o	**-rrhexis**
		-stenosis
		-ectomy

5.81. Inflammation of an artery or arteries is known as _____.

5.82. The surgical removal of a portion of a blood vessel is a/an _____.

5.83. The abnormal narrowing of the lumen of a vein is known as _____.

5.84. The surgical removal of a portion of the tissue surrounding the heart is a/an _____.

5.85. To surgically suture the wall of the heart is a/an _____.

5.86. Rupture of a vein is known as _____.

5.87. The suture repair of any vessel, especially a blood vessel, is a/an _____.

5.88. Rupture of the heart is known as _____.

5.89. To suture the tissue surrounding the heart is a/an _____.

5.90. The tissue death of the walls of the blood vessels is known as _____.

Labeling Exercises

Identify the numbered items in the accompanying figures.

5.91. superior _____

5.92. right _____

5.93. right _____

5.94. left pulmonary _____

5.95. left pulmonary _____

5.96. pulmonary _____ valve

5.97. _____ valve

5.98. _____

5.99. _____ semilunar valve

5.100. _____ valve

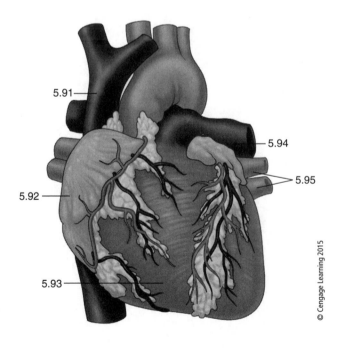

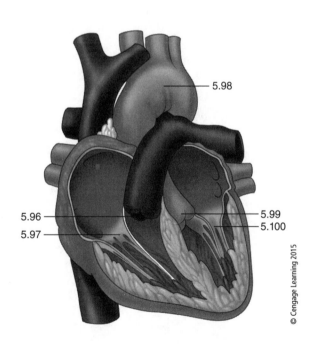

© Cengage Learning 2015

CHAPTER 6

The Lymphatic and Immune Systems

Learning Exercises

Class _____   Name _____

Matching Word Parts 1

Write the correct answer in the middle column.

Definition	Correct Answer	Possible Answers
6.1. against	_____	**anti-**
6.2. eat, swallow	_____	**lymphaden/o**
6.3. lymph node	_____	**lymphangi/o**
6.4. lymph vessel	_____	**phag/o**
6.5. poison	_____	**tox/o**

Matching Word Parts 2

Write the correct answer in the middle column.

Definition	Correct Answer	Possible Answers
6.6. flesh	_____	**immun/o**
6.7. formative material of cells	_____	**onc/o**
6.8. protection, safe	_____	**-plasm**
6.9. spleen	_____	**sarc/o**
6.10. tumor	_____	**splen/o**

Matching Types of Pathogens

Write the correct answer in the middle column.

Definition	Correct Answer	Possible Answers
6.11. bacteria capable of movement	_____	parasites
6.12. chain-forming bacteria	_____	spirochetes
6.13. cluster-forming bacteria	_____	staphylococci
6.14. live only by invading cells	_____	streptococci
6.15. live within other organisms	_____	viruses

Definitions

Select the correct answer, and write it on the line provided.

6.16. The _____ has/have a hemolytic function.

    appendix   lymph nodes   spleen   tonsils

6.17. Inflammation of the lymph nodes is known as _____.

    angiogenesis   lymphadenitis   lymphedema   lymphoma

6.18. The medical term for the condition commonly known as shingles is _____.

    cytomegalovirus   herpes zoster   rubella   varicella

6.19. Proteins that activate the immune system, fight viruses by slowing or stopping their multiplication, and signal other cells to increase their defenses are known as _____.

    T cells   immunoglobulins   interferons   synthetic immunoglobulins

6.20. The _____ plays specialized roles in both the lymphatic and immune systems.

    bone marrow   liver   spleen   thymus

6.21. The protective ring of lymphoid tissue around the back of the nose and upper throat is formed by the _____.

    lacteals   lymph nodes   tonsils   villi

6.22. Secondary _____ can be caused by cancer treatments, burns, or injuries.

    lymphadenitis   lymphangioma   lymphadenopathy   lymphedema

6.23. Fats that cannot be transported by the bloodstream are absorbed by the _____ that are located in the villi that line the small intestine.

    lacteals   lymph nodes   B cells   spleen

6.24. The parasite _____ is most commonly transmitted from pets to humans by contact with contaminated animal feces.

    herpes zoster   malaria   rabies   toxoplasmosis

6.25. A _____ is a type of leukocyte that surrounds and kills invading cells. This type of cell also removes dead cells and stimulates the action of other immune cells.

    B lymphocyte   macrophage   platelet   T lymphocyte

Matching Structures

Write the correct answer in the middle column.

Definition	Correct Answer	Possible Answers
6.26. filter harmful substances from lymph	_____	complement system cells
6.27. lymphoid tissue hanging from the lower portion of the cecum	_____	intact skin
6.28. combine with antibodies to dissolve foreign cells	_____	lymph nodes
6.29. stores extra erythrocytes	_____	spleen
6.30. wraps the body in a physical barrier	_____	vermiform appendix

Which Word?

Select the correct answer, and write it on the line provided.

6.31. The _____ act as intracellular signals to begin the immune response.

cytokines   macrophages

6.32. A _____ drug is a medication that kills or damages cells.

corticosteroid   cytotoxic

6.33. The _____ develop from B cells and secrete large bodies of antibodies coded to destroy specific antigens.

Reed-Sternberg cells   plasma cells

6.34. The antibody therapy known as _____ is used to treat multiple sclerosis, hepatitis C, and some cancers.

monoclonal antibodies   synthetic interferon

6.35. Infectious mononucleosis is caused by a _____.

spirochete   virus

Spelling Counts

Find the misspelled word in each sentence. Then write that word, spelled correctly, on the line provided.

6.36. A sarkoma is a malignant tumor that arises from connective tissue. _____

6.37. The adanoids, which are also known as the nasopharyngeal tonsils, are located in the nasopharynx. _____

6.38. Lymphiscintigraphy is a diagnostic test that is performed to detect damage or malformations of the lymphatic vessels. _____

6.39. Antiobiotics are commonly used to combat bacterial infections. _____

6.40. Varichella is commonly known as chickenpox. _____

Abbreviation Identification

In the space provided, write the words that each abbreviation stands for.

6.41. CIS _____

6.42. DCIS _____

6.43. LE _____

6.44. MMR _____

6.45. Ag _____

Term Selection

Select the correct answer, and write it on the line provided.

6.46. _____ is the process through which a tumor supports its growth by creating its own blood supply.

metastasis   angiogenesis   neoplasm   malignant tumor

6.47. An opportunistic infection that is frequently associated with HIV is _____.

Hodgkin's disease   Kaposi's sarcoma   myasthenia gravis   tinea pedis

6.48. Malaria is caused by a _____ that is transferred to humans by the bite of an infected mosquito.

parasite   rickettsiae   spirochete   virus

6.49. Bacilli, which are rod-shaped, spore-forming bacteria, cause _____.

Lyme disease   measles   rubella   anthrax

6.50. Swelling of the parotid glands is a symptom of _____.

measles   mumps   shingles   rubella

Sentence Completion

Write the correct term or terms on the lines provided.

6.51. A severe systemic reaction to an allergen causing serious symptoms that develop very quickly is known as _____.

6.52. In _____, radioactive materials are implanted into the tissues to be treated.

6.53. When testing for HIV, a/an _____ test produces more accurate results than the ELISA test.

6.54. A/An _____ is a benign tumor formed by an abnormal collection of lymphatic vessels.

6.55. After primary cancer treatments have been completed, _____ therapy is used to decrease the chances that the cancer will recur.

Word Surgery

Divide each term into its component word parts. Write these word parts, in sequence, on the lines provided. When necessary, use a slash (/) to indicate a combining vowel. (You may not need all of the lines provided.)

6.56. An **antineoplastic** is a medication that blocks the development, growth, or proliferation of malignant cells.

_____ _____ _____ _____

6.57. **Metastasis** is the new cancer site that results from the spreading process.

_____ _____ _____ _____

6.58. **Osteosarcoma** is a hard-tissue sarcoma that usually involves the upper shaft of the long bones, pelvis, or knee.

_____ _____ _____ _____

6.59. **Cytomegalovirus** is a member of the *herpesvirus* family that causes a variety of diseases.

_____ _____ _____ _____

6.60. **Antiangiogenesis** is a form of cancer treatment that disrupts the blood supply to the tumor.

_____ _____ _____ _____

True/False

If the statement is true, write **True** on the line. If the statement is false, write **False** on the line.

6.61. _____ Inflammatory breast cancer is the most aggressive and least common form of breast cancer.

6.62. _____ Lymph carries nutrients and oxygen to the cells.

6.63. _____ A myosarcoma is a benign tumor derived from muscle tissue.

6.64. _____ Reed-Sternberg cells are present in Hodgkin's lymphoma.

6.65. _____ Septic shock is caused by a viral infection.

Clinical Conditions

Write the correct answer on the line provided.

6.66. Dr. Wei diagnosed her patient as having an enlarged spleen due to damage caused by his injuries. The medical term for this condition is _____.

6.67. At the beginning of the treatment of Juanita Phillips' breast cancer, a/an _____ breast biopsy was performed using an x-ray-guided needle.

6.68. Mr. Grossman described his serious illness as being caused by a "superbug infection." His doctor describes these bacteria as being _____.

6.69. Dorothy Peterson was diagnosed with breast cancer. She and her doctor agreed upon treating this surgically with a/an _____. This is a procedure in which the cancerous tissue with a margin of normal tissue is removed.

6.70. Every day since his kidney transplant, Mr. Lanning must take a/an _____ to prevent rejection of the donor organ.

6.71. Rosita Sanchez is 2 months pregnant, and she and her doctor are worried because her rash was diagnosed as _____. They are concerned because this condition can produce defects in Rosita's developing child.

6.72. Tarana Inglis took _____ to relieve the symptoms of her allergies.

6.73. The _____ virus is spread to humans through the bite of an infected mosquito. The more severe variety spreads to the spinal cord and brain.

6.74. John Fogelman was diagnosed with having a/an _____. This is a malignant tumor that arises from connective tissues, including hard, soft, and liquid tissues.

6.75. Jane Doe is infected with HIV. One of her medications is acyclovir, which is a/an _____ drug.

Which Is the Correct Medical Term?

Select the correct answer, and write it on the line provided.

6.76. The _____ are specialized lymphocytes that produce antibodies. Each lymphocyte makes a specific antibody that is capable of destroying a specific antigen.

B cells   bacilli   immunoglobulins   T cells

6.77. Any of a large group of diseases characterized by a condition in which the immune system produces antibodies against its own tissues is known as a/an _____ disorder.

autoimmune   allergy   rubella   immunodeficiency

6.78. The _____ lymph nodes are located in the groin.

axillary   cervical   inguinal   subcutaneous

6.79. A/An _____ is any one of a large group of carcinomas derived from glandular tissue.

adenocarcinoma   lymphoma   myosarcoma   myoma

6.80. A/An _____ drug is used either as an immunosuppressant or as an antineoplastic.

corticosteroid   cytotoxic   immunoglobulin   monoclonal

Challenge Word Building

These terms are *not* found in this chapter; however, they are made up of the following familiar word parts. If you need help in creating the term, refer to your medical dictionary.

adenoid/o	**-ectomy**
lymphaden/o	**-itis**
lymphang/o	**-ology**
immun/o	**-oma**
splen/o	**-rrhaphy**
tonsill/o	
thym/o	

6.81. The study of the immune system is known as _____.

6.82. Surgical removal of the spleen is a/an _____.

6.83. Inflammation of the thymus is known as _____.

6.84. Inflammation of the lymph vessels is known as _____.

6.85. The term meaning to suture the spleen is _____.

6.86. The surgical removal of the adenoids is a/an _____.

6.87. The surgical removal of a lymph node is a/an _____.

6.88. A tumor originating in the thymus is known as _____.

6.89. Inflammation of the tonsils is known as _____.

6.90. Inflammation of the spleen is known as _____.

Labeling Exercises

Identify the numbered items on the accompanying figures.

6.91. tonsils and _____

6.92. Lymphocytes are formed in bone _____

6.93. large intestine and _____

6.94. _____

6.95. _____

6.96. _____ lymph nodes

6.97. Right _____ empties into the right subclavian vein.

6.98. _____ duct

6.99. _____ lymph nodes

6.100. _____ lymph nodes

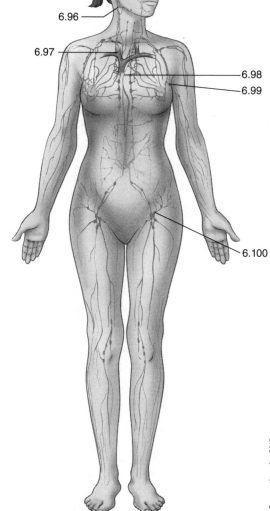

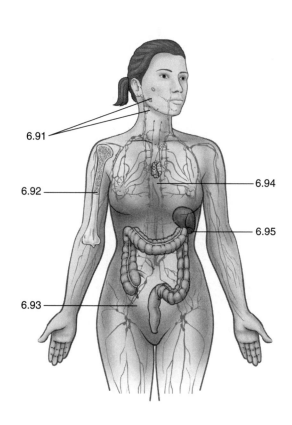

The Respiratory System

Learning Exercises

Class _____   Name _____

Matching Word Parts 1

Write the correct answer in the middle column.

Definition	Correct Answer	Possible Answers
7.1. nose	_____	**nas/o**
7.2. sleep	_____	**laryng/o**
7.3. to breathe	_____	**pharyng/o**
7.4. throat, pharynx	_____	**somn/o**
7.5. larynx, throat	_____	**spir/o**

Matching Word Parts 2

Write the correct answer in the middle column.

Definition	Correct Answer	Possible Answers
7.6. lung	_____	**bronch/o**
7.7. oxygen	_____	**ox/o**
7.8. pleura	_____	**phon/o**
7.9. bronchus	_____	**pleur/o**
7.10. sound or voice	_____	**pneum/o**

Matching Word Parts 3

Write the correct answer in the middle column.

Definition	Correct Answer	Possible Answers
7.11. windpipe	_____	**-pnea**
7.12. sinus	_____	**pulmon/o**
7.13. lung	_____	**sinus/o**
7.14. chest	_____	**-thorax**
7.15. breathing	_____	**trache/o**

Definitions

Select the correct answer, and write it on the line provided.

7.16. The heart, aorta, esophagus, and trachea are located in the _____.

    dorsal cavity   manubrium   mediastinum   pleura

7.17. The _____ acts as a lid over the entrance to the laryngopharynx.

    Adam's apple   epiglottis   larynx   thyroid cartilage

7.18. The innermost layer of the pleura is known as the _____.

    parietal pleura   pleural space   pleural cavity   visceral pleura

7.19. The _____ sinuses are located just above the eyebrows.

    ethmoid   frontal   maxillary   sphenoid

7.20. The smallest divisions of the bronchial tree are the _____.

    alveoli   alveolus   bronchioles   bronchi

7.21. During respiration, the exchange of oxygen and carbon dioxide takes place through the walls of the _____.

    alveoli   arteries   capillaries   veins

7.22. The term meaning spitting blood or blood-stained sputum is _____.

    effusion   epistaxis   hemoptysis   hemothorax

7.23. Black lung disease is the lay term for _____.

    anthracosis   asbestosis   pneumoconiosis   silicosis

7.24. The term _____ means an abnormally rapid rate of respiration.

    apnea   bradypnea   dyspnea   tachypnea

7.25. The term meaning any voice impairment is _____.

    aphonia   dysphonia   laryngitis   laryngospasm

Matching Structures

Write the correct answer in the middle column.

Definition	Correct Answer	Possible Answers
7.26. first division of the pharynx	_____	**laryngopharynx**
7.27. second division of the pharynx	_____	**larynx**
7.28. third division of the pharynx	_____	**nasopharynx**
7.29. voice box	_____	**oropharynx**
7.30. windpipe	_____	**trachea**

Which Word?

Select the correct answer, and write it on the line provided.

7.31. The exchange of gases within the cells of the body is known as _____.

    external respiration   internal respiration

7.32. The term that describes the lung disease caused by asbestos particles in the lungs is _____.

    asbestosis   silicosis

7.33. The form of pneumonia that can be prevented through vaccination is _____.

    bacterial pneumonia   viral pneumonia

7.34. The term commonly known as shortness of breath is _____.

    dyspnea   eupnea

7.35. The emergency procedure to gain access below a blocked airway is known as a _____.

    tracheostomy   tracheotomy

Spelling Counts

Find the misspelled word in each sentence. Then write the word, spelled correctly, on the line provided.

7.36. The thick mucus secreted by the tissues that line the respiratory passages is called phlem. _____

7.37. The medical term meaning an accumulation of pus in a body cavity is empiema. _____

7.38. The medical name for the disease commonly known as whooping cough is pertusis. _____

7.39. The frenic nerves stimulate the diaphragm and cause it to contract. _____

7.40. An antitussiff is administered to prevent or relieve coughing. _____

Abbreviation Identification

In the space provided, write the words that each abbreviation stands for.

7.41. **ARDS** _____

7.42. **CF** _____

7.43. **FESS** _____

7.44. **SIDS** _____

7.45. **URI** _____

Term Selection

Select the correct answer, and write it on the line provided.

7.46. Inhaling a foreign substance into the upper respiratory tract can cause _____ pneumonia.

aspiration   inhalation   inspiration   respiration

7.47. The term meaning abnormally rapid deep breathing is _____.

dyspnea   hyperpnea   hypopnea   hyperventilation

7.48. The term meaning the surgical creation of a stoma into the trachea to insert a breathing tube is _____.

bronchiectasis   thoracotomy   tracheostomy   tracheotomy

7.49. The diaphragm is relaxed during _____.

exhalation   inhalation   internal respiration   singultus

7.50. The chronic allergic disorder characterized by episodes of severe breathing difficulty, coughing, and wheezing is known as _____.

allergic rhinitis   asthma   bronchospasm   laryngospasm

Sentence Completion

Write the correct term or terms on the lines provided.

7.51. The term meaning an absence of spontaneous respiration is _____.

7.52. The sudden spasmodic closure of the larynx is a/an _____.

7.53. The term meaning bleeding from the lungs is _____.

7.54. The term meaning pain in the pleura or in the side is _____.

7.55. A contraction of the smooth muscle in the walls of the bronchi and bronchioles that tighten and squeeze the airway shut is known as a/an _____.

Word Surgery

Divide each term into its component word parts. Write these word parts, in sequence, on the lines provided. When necessary, use a slash (/) to indicate a combining vowel. (You may not need all of the lines provided.)

7.56. **Bronchorrhea** means an excessive discharge of mucus from the bronchi.

_____   _____   _____   _____

7.57. The **oropharynx** is visible when looking at the back of the mouth.

_____   _____   _____   _____

7.58. **Polysomnography** measures physiological activity during sleep and is most often performed to detect nocturnal defects in breathing associated with sleep apnea.

_____   _____   _____   _____

7.59. **Pneumorrhagia** is bleeding from the lungs.

_____   _____   _____   _____

7.60. **Rhinorrhea**, also known as a runny nose, is an excessive flow of mucus from the nose.

_____   _____   _____   _____

True/False

If the statement is true, write **True** on the line. If the statement is false, write **False** on the line.

7.61. _____ A pulse oximeter is a monitor placed inside the ear to measure the oxygen saturation level in the blood.

7.62. _____ In atelectasis, the lung fails to expand because there is a blockage of the air passages or pneumothorax.

7.63. _____ Croup is an allergic reaction to airborne allergens.

7.64. _____ Hypoxemia is the condition of below-normal oxygenation of arterial blood.

7.65. _____ Emphysema is the progressive loss of lung function in which the chest sometimes assumes an enlarged barrel shape.

Clinical Conditions

Write the correct answer on the line provided.

7.66. Baby Jamison was born with _____. This is a genetic disorder in which the lungs are clogged with large quantities of abnormally thick mucus.

7.67. Dr. Lee surgically removed a portion of the lung. This procedure is known as a/an
_____.

7.68. Wendy Barlow required the surgical removal of her larynx. This procedure is known as a/an
_____.

7.69. During his asthma attacks, Jamaal Nelson uses an inhaler containing a _____. This medication expands the opening of the passages into his lungs.

7.70. Each year, Mr. Partin receives a flu shot to prevent _____.

7.71. When hit during a fight, Marvin Roper's nose started to bleed. The medical term for this condition is _____.

7.72. The doctor's examination revealed that Juanita Martinez has an accumulation of blood in the pleural cavity. This diagnosis is recorded on her chart as a/an _____.

7.73. Duncan McClanahan had a/an _____ performed to correct damage to the septum of his nose.

7.74. Suzanne Holderman is suffering from an inflammation of the bronchial walls. The medical term for Suzanne's condition is chronic _____.

7.75. Ted Coleman required the permanent placement of a breathing tube. The procedure for the placement of this tube is called a/an _____.

Which Is the Correct Medical Term?

Select the correct answer, and write it on the line provided.

7.76. An inflammation of the pleura that causes pleurodynia is known as _____.

atelectasis   emphysema   pleurodynia   pleurisy

7.77. The substance ejected through the mouth and used for diagnostic purposes in respiratory disorders is known as _____.

phlegm   pleural effusion   saliva   sputum

7.78. The term meaning a bluish discoloration of the skin caused by a lack of adequate oxygen is _____.

asphyxia   cyanosis   epistaxis   hypoxia

7.79. The medical term meaning sudden spasmodic closure of the larynx is _____.

aphonia   dysphonia   laryngitis   laryngospasm

7.80. The pattern of alternating periods of rapid breathing, slow breathing, and the absence of breathing is known as _____.

anoxia   Cheyne-Stokes respiration   eupnea   tachypnea

Challenge Word Building

These terms are *not* found in this chapter; however, they are made up of the following familiar word parts. If you need help in creating the term, refer to your medical dictionary.

bronch/o	**-itis**
epiglott/o	**-ologist**
laryng/o	**-plasty**
pharyng/o	**-plegia**
pneumon/o	**-rrhagia**
trache/o	**-rrhea**
	-scopy
	-stenosis

7.81. An abnormal discharge from the pharynx is known as _____.

7.82. Inflammation of the lungs is known as _____.

7.83. A specialist in the study of the larynx is a/an _____.

7.84. Bleeding from the larynx is known as _____.

7.85. Inflammation of both the pharynx and the larynx is known as _____.

7.86. Abnormal narrowing of the lumen of the trachea is known as _____.

7.87. The surgical repair of a bronchial defect is a/an _____.

7.88. Inflammation of the epiglottis is known as _____.

7.89. The inspection of both the trachea and bronchi through a bronchoscope is a/an _____.

7.90. Paralysis of the walls of the bronchi is known as _____.

Labeling Exercises

Identify the parts of numbered items on the accompanying figure.

7.91. _____

7.92. _____

7.93. _____

7.94. _____

7.95. _____

7.96. _____ cavity

7.97. _____

7.98. _____

7.99. _____ lung

7.100. _____ sacs

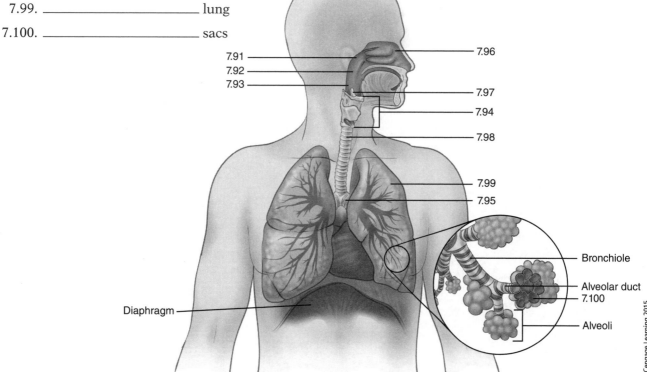

Diaphragm

Bronchiole

Alveolar duct

7.100

Alveoli

© Cengage Learning 2015

CHAPTER 8

The Digestive System

Learning Exercises

Class _____   Name _____

Matching Word Parts 1

Write the correct answer in the middle column.

Definition	Correct Answer	Possible Answers
8.1. anus	_____	**chol/e**
8.2. bile, gall	_____	**an/o**
8.3. large intestine	_____	**col/o**
8.4. swallowing	_____	**enter/o**
8.5. small intestine	_____	**-phagia**

Matching Word Parts 2

Write the correct answer in the middle column.

Definition	Correct Answer	Possible Answers
8.6. stomach	_____	**cholecyst/o**
8.7. liver	_____	**esophag/o**
8.8. gallbladder	_____	**gastr/o**
8.9. esophagus	_____	**hepat/o**
8.10. presence of stones	_____	**-lithiasis**

Matching Word Parts 3

Write the correct answer in the middle column.

Definition	Correct Answer	Possible Answers
8.11. sigmoid colon	_____	**-pepsia**
8.12. anus and rectum	_____	**-emesis**
8.13. digestion	_____	**proct/o**
8.14. vomiting	_____	**rect/o**
8.15. rectum	_____	**sigmoid/o**

Definitions

Select the correct answer, and write it on the line provided.

8.16. The visual examination of the anal canal and lower rectum is known as _____.

anoscopy   colonoscopy   proctoscopy   sigmoidoscopy

8.17. The term _____ means any disease of the mouth due to a fungus.

salmonellosis   stomatomycosis   stomatitis   steatorrhea

8.18. The _____ is the last and longest portion of the small intestine.

cecum   ileum   jejunum   pylorus

8.19. The inability to control the excretion of feces is called _____.

bowel incontinence   constipation   anal fissure   hematochezia

8.20. The liver secretes _____, which is stored in the gallbladder for later use.

bile   glycogen   insulin   pepsin

8.21. The _____ travels upward from the cecum to the undersurface of the liver.

ascending colon   descending colon   sigmoid colon   transverse colon

8.22. The process of the building up of body cells and substances from nutrients is known as

_____.

anabolism   catabolism   defecation   mastication

8.23. The receptors of taste are located on the dorsum of the _____.

hard palate   rugae   tongue   uvula

8.24. The bone and soft tissues that surround and support the teeth are known as the

_____.

dentition   gingiva   occlusion   periodontium

8.25. The condition characterized by the telescoping of one part of the intestine into another is

_____.

borborygmus   flatus   intussusception   volvulus

Matching Structures

Write the correct answer in the middle column.

Definition	Correct Answer	Possible Answers
8.26. connects the small and large intestine	_____	cecum
8.27. S-shaped structure of the large intestine	_____	duodenum
8.28. widest division of the large intestine	_____	jejunum
8.29. middle portion of the small intestine	_____	rectum
8.30. first portion of the small intestine	_____	sigmoid colon

Which Word?

Select the correct answer, and write it on the line provided.

8.31. The medical term meaning vomiting blood is _____.

    hematemesis   hyperemesis

8.32. The _____ virus is transmitted mainly through contamination of food and water with infected fecal matter.

    hepatitis A   hepatitis B

8.33. _____ is characterized by a severe reaction to foods containing gluten.

    celiac disease   Crohn's disease

8.34. The medical term meaning inflammation of the small intestine is _____.

    colitis   enteritis

8.35. The _____ hangs from the free edge of the soft palate.

    rugae   uvula

Spelling Counts

Find the misspelled word in each sentence. Then write that word, spelled correctly, on the line provided.

8.36. An ilectomy is the surgical removal of the last portion of the ileum. _____

8.37. The bacterial infection disentary occurs mostly in hot countries and is spread through food or water contaminated by human feces. _____

8.38. The chronic degenerative disease of the liver characterized by scarring is known as serosis. _____

8.39. A proctoplexy is the surgical fixation of the rectum to some adjacent tissue or organ. _____

8.40. The lack of adequate saliva due to the absence of or diminished secretions by the salivary glands is known as zerostomia. _____

Abbreviation Identification

In the space provided, write the words that each abbreviation stands for.

8.41. **UC** _____

8.42. **COL** _____

8.43. **GERD** _____

8.44. **IBS** _____

8.45. **PUD** _____

Term Selection

Select the correct answer, and write it on the line provided.

8.46. The surgical removal of all or part of the stomach is a _____.

gastrectomy   gastritis   gastroenteritis   gastrotomy

8.47. The medical term meaning difficulty in swallowing is _____.

anorexia   dyspepsia   dysphagia   pyrosis

8.48. The involuntary grinding or clenching of the teeth is called _____.

bruxism   edentulous   malocclusion   dental caries

8.49. The chronic degeneration of the liver often caused by excessive alcohol abuse is called

_____.

cirrhosis   hepatitis C   hepatitis A   hepatomegaly

8.50. Jaundice can be caused by an excess of the pigment called _____.

bile   bilirubin   hydrochloric acid   pancreatic juice

Sentence Completion

Write the correct term or terms on the lines provided.

8.51. The excessive swallowing of air while eating or drinking is known as _____.

8.52. The return of swallowed food to the mouth is known as _____.

8.53. A yellow discoloration of the skin caused by greater-than-normal amounts of bilirubin in the blood is called _____.

8.54. The _____ is the ring-like muscle that controls the flow from the stomach to the small intestine.

8.55. The medical term for the solid body wastes that are expelled through the rectum is _____.

Word Surgery

Divide each term into its component word parts. Write these word parts, in sequence, on the lines provided. When necessary use a slash (/) to indicate a combining vowel. (You may not need all of the lines provided.)

8.56. An **esophagogastroduodenoscopy** is an endoscopic procedure that allows direct visualization of the upper GI tract.

_____ _____ _____ _____

8.57. A **periodontist** is a dental specialist who prevents or treats disorders of the tissues surrounding the teeth.

_____ _____ _____ _____

8.58. A **sigmoidoscopy** is the endoscopic examination of the interior of the rectum, sigmoid colon, and possibly a portion of the descending colon.

_____ _____ _____ _____

8.59. An **antiemetic** is a medication that is administered to prevent or relieve nausea and vomiting.

_____ _____ _____ _____

8.60. A **gastroduodenostomy** is the establishment of an anastomosis between the upper portion of the stomach and the duodenum.

_____ _____ _____ _____

True/False

If the statement is true, write **True** on the line. If the statement is false, write **False** on the line.

8.61. _____ Cholangitis is an acute infection of the bile duct characterized by pain in the upper right quadrant of the abdomen, fever, and jaundice.

8.62. _____ Cholangiography is an endoscopic diagnostic procedure.

8.63. _____ Acute necrotizing ulcerative gingivitis is caused by the abnormal growth of bacteria in the mouth.

8.64. _____ Bruxism means to be without natural teeth.

8.65. _____ A choledocholithotomy is an incision in the common bile duct for the removal of gallstones.

Clinical Conditions

Write the correct answer on the line provided.

8.66. James Ridgeview was diagnosed as having _____, which is the partial or complete blockage of the small or large intestine.

8.67. Chang Hoon suffers from _____. This condition is an abnormal accumulation of serous fluid in the peritoneal cavity.

8.68. Rita Martinez is a dentist. She described her patient Mr. Espinoza as being _____, which means that he was without natural teeth.

8.69. Baby Kilgore was vomiting almost continuously. The medical term for this excessive vomiting is _____.

8.70. A/An _____ was performed on Mr. Schmidt to create an artificial excretory opening between his colon and body surface.

8.71. After eating, Mike Delahanty often complained about heartburn. The medical term for this condition is _____.

8.72. After the repeated passage of black, tarry, and foul-smelling stools, Catherine Baldwin was diagnosed as having _____. This condition is caused by the presence of digested blood in the stools.

8.73. Alberta Roberts was diagnosed as having an inflammation of one or more diverticula. The medical term for this condition is _____.

8.74. Carlotta Hansen has blister-like sores on her lips and adjacent facial tissue. She says they are cold sores; however, the medical term for this condition is _____ .

8.75. Lisa Wilson saw her dentist because she was concerned about bad breath. Her dentist refers to this condition as _____.

Which Is the Correct Medical Term?

Select the correct answer, and write it on the line provided.

8.76. The _____ test detects hidden blood in the stools.

| anoscopy | colonoscopy | enema | Hemoccult |

8.77. A/An _____ is a surgical connection between two hollow or tubular structures.

| anastomosis | ostomy | stoma | sphincter |

8.78. The eating disorder characterized by voluntary starvation and excessive exercising because of an intense fear of gaining weight is known as _____.

| anorexia | anorexia nervosa | bulimia | bulimia nervosa |

8.79. The hardened deposit that forms on the teeth and irritates the surrounding tissues is known as dental _____.

| calculus | caries | decay | plaque |

8.80. The surgical removal of all or part of the liver is known as _____.

| anoplasty | palatoplasty | proctopexy | hepatectomy |

Challenge Word Building

These terms are *not* found in this chapter; however, they are made up of the following familiar word parts. If you need help in creating the term, refer to your medical dictionary.

col/o	-algia
enter/o	-ectomy
esophag/o	-ic
gastr/o	-itis
hepat/o	-megaly
proct/o	-pexy
sigmoid/o	-rrhaphy

8.81. Surgical suturing of a stomach wound is known as _____.

8.82. Pain in the esophagus is known as _____.

8.83. The surgical removal of all or part of the sigmoid colon is a/an _____.

8.84. Pain in and around the anus and rectum is known as _____.

8.85. The surgical fixation of the stomach to correct displacement is a/an _____.

8.86. Inflammation of the sigmoid colon is known as _____.

8.87. The surgical removal of all or part of the esophagus and stomach is a/an _____.

8.88. The term meaning relating to the liver and intestines is _____.

8.89. Abnormal enlargement of the liver is known as _____.

8.90. Inflammation of the stomach, small intestine, and colon is known as _____.

Labeling Exercises

Identify the numbered items on the accompanying figure.

8.91. _____ glands

8.92. _____

8.93. _____

8.94. _____

8.95. _____

8.96. _____

8.97. _____ intestine

8.98. vermiform _____

8.99. _____ intestine

8.100. _____ and anus

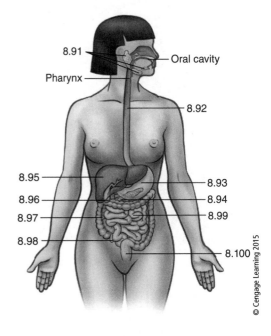

The Urinary System

Learning Exercises

Class _____   Name _____

Matching Word Parts 1

Write the correct answer in the middle column.

Definition	Correct Answer	Possible Answers
9.1. bladder	_____	**-cele**
9.2. glomerulus	_____	**cyst/o**
9.3. hernia, tumor, cyst	_____	**glomerul/o**
9.4. kidney	_____	**lith/o**
9.5. stone, calculus	_____	**nephr/o**

Matching Word Parts 2

Write the correct answer in the middle column.

Definition	Correct Answer	Possible Answers
9.6. urine, urinary tract	_____	**-tripsy**
9.7. renal pelvis	_____	**pyel/o**
9.8. setting free, separation	_____	**ur/o**
9.9. surgical fixation	_____	**-pexy**
9.10. to crush	_____	**-lysis**

Matching Word Parts 3

Write the correct answer in the middle column.

Definition	Correct Answer	Possible Answers
9.11. complete, through	_____	**-uria**
9.12. enlargement, stretching	_____	**urethr/o**
9.13. ureter	_____	**ureter/o**
9.14. urethra	_____	**-ectasis**
9.15. urination, urine	_____	**dia-**

Definitions

Select the correct answer, and write it on the line provided.

9.16. Urine is carried from the kidneys to the urinary bladder by the _____.

    glomeruli   nephrons   urethras   ureters

9.17. A stone in the urinary bladder is known as a _____.

    cholelith   cystolith   nephrolith   ureterolith

9.18. The increased output of urine is known as _____.

    anuria   diuresis   dysuria   oliguria

9.19. Before entering the ureters, urine collects in the _____.

    glomeruli   renal cortex   renal pelvis   urinary bladder

9.20. Urine leaves the bladder through the _____.

    prostate   kidney   ureter   urethra

9.21. Urine is produced in microscopic functional units of each kidney called _____.

    uremia   ureters   urethra   nephrons

9.22. In the male, the _____ carries both urine and semen.

    prostate gland   renal pelvis   ureter   urethra

9.23. A specialist who treats the genitourinary system of males is a/an _____.

    gynecologist   nephrologist   neurologist   urologist

9.24. In _____, the urethral opening is on the upper surface of the penis.

    epispadias   hyperspadias   hypospadias   urethritis

9.25. The term _____ describes treatment in which a body part is removed or its function is destroyed. This type of procedure is frequently used to treat prostate cancer.

    ablation   adhesion   lithotomy   meatotomy

Matching Structures

Write the correct answer in the middle column.

Definition	Correct Answer	Possible Answers
9.26. the opening through which urine leaves the body	_____	urethral meatus
9.27. the portion of a nephron that is active in filtering urine	_____	urethra
9.28. the outer region of the kidney	_____	ureters
9.29. the tube from the bladder to the outside of the body	_____	renal cortex
9.30. the tubes that carry urine from the kidney to the bladder	_____	glomerulus

Which Word?

Select the correct answer, and write it on the line provided.

9.31. A surgical incision into the renal pelvis is a _____.

      pyelotomy   pyeloplasty

9.32. The discharge of blood from the ureter is _____.

      ureterorrhagia   urethrorrhagia

9.33. The term meaning excessive urination is _____.

      incontinence   polyuria

9.34. The term meaning inflammation of the bladder is _____.

      cystitis   pyelitis

9.35. The major waste product of protein metabolism is _____.

      urea   urine

Spelling Counts

Find the misspelled word in each sentence. Then write that word, spelled correctly, on the line provided.

9.36. A Willms tumor is a malignant tumor of the kidney that occurs in children.

_____

9.37. Being unable to control excretory functions is known as incontinance. _____

9.38. The process of withdrawing urine from the bladder is known as urinary cathaterization.

_____

9.39. Keagel exercises are a series of pelvic muscle exercises used to strengthen the muscles of the pelvic floor to control urinary stress incontinence. _____

9.40. A vesicovaginel fistula is an abnormal opening between the bladder and vagina.

_____

Abbreviation Identification

In the space provided, write the words that each abbreviation stands for.

9.41. **BPH** _____

9.42. **ESRD** _____

9.43. **ESWL** _____

9.44. **IVP** _____

9.45. **OAB** _____

Term Selection

Select the correct answer, and write it on the line provided.

9.46. The absence of urine formation by the kidneys is known as _____.

anuria   nocturia   oliguria   polyuria

9.47. The surgical suturing of the bladder is known as _____.

cystorrhaphy   cystorrhagia   cystorrhexis   nephrorrhaphy

9.48. The term meaning the freeing of a kidney from adhesions is _____.

nephrolithiasis   nephrolysis   anuria   pyelitis

9.49. The term meaning scanty urination is _____.

diuresis   dysuria   enuresis   oliguria

9.50. The process of artificially filtering waste products from the patient's blood is known as _____.

diuresis   hemodialysis   homeostasis   hydroureter

Sentence Completion

Write the correct term or terms on the lines provided.

9.51. An inflammation of the kidney, most commonly caused by toxins, infection, or an autoimmune disease is called _____.

9.52. A stone located anywhere along the ureter is known as a _____.

9.53. The placement of a catheter into the bladder through a small incision made through the abdominal wall just above the pubic bone is known as _____.

9.54. The surgical fixation of the bladder to the abdominal wall is a/an _____.

9.55. A/An _____ (TURP) is the removal of excess tissue from the prostate with the use of a resectoscope.

Word Surgery

Divide each term into its component word parts. Write these word parts, in sequence, on the lines provided. When necessary, use a slash (/) to indicate a combining vowel. (You may not need all of the lines provided.)

9.56. **Hyperproteinuria** is abnormally high concentrations of protein in the urine.

_____   _____   _____   _____

9.57. **Hydronephrosis** is the dilation of one or both kidneys.

_____   _____   _____   _____

9.58. Voiding **cystourethrography** is a diagnostic procedure in which a fluoroscope is used to examine the flow of urine from the bladder and through the urethra.

_____   _____   _____   _____

9.59. A percutaneous **nephrolithotomy** is the surgical removal of a kidney stone through a small incision in the back.

_____   _____   _____   _____

9.60. **Ureterorrhaphy** means the surgical suturing of a ureter.

_____   _____   _____   _____

True/False

If the statement is true, write **True** on the line. If the statement is false, write **False** on the line.

9.61. _____ Stress incontinence is the inability to control the voiding of urine under physical stress such as running, sneezing, laughing, or coughing.

9.62. _____ Prostatism is a malignancy of the prostate gland.

9.63. _____ Urethrorrhea is bleeding from the urethra.

9.64. _____ Renal colic is an acute pain in the kidney area that is caused by blockage during the passage of a kidney stone.

9.65. _____ Acute renal failure has sudden onset and is characterized by uremia.

Clinical Conditions

Write the correct answer on the line provided.

9.66. Mr. Baldridge suffers from excessive urination during the night. The medical term for this is _____.

9.67. Rosita LaPinta inherited _____ kidney disease. These cysts slowly reduce the kidney function, and this eventually leads to kidney failure.

9.68. Doris Volk has a chronic bladder condition involving inflammation within the wall of the bladder. This is known as _____.

9.69. John Danielson has an enlarged prostate gland. This caused narrowing of the urethra, which is known as _____.

9.70. Norman Smith was born with the opening of the urethra on the upper surface of the penis. This is known as _____.

9.71. Henry Wong's kidneys failed. He is being treated with _____, which involves the removal of waste from his blood through a fluid exchange in the abdominal cavity.

9.72. Roberta Gridley is scheduled for surgical repair of damage to the ureter. This procedure is a/an _____.

9.73. When Lenny Nowicki's _____ blood test showed a very high PSA level, his physician was concerned about the possibility of prostate cancer.

9.74. Dr. Morita's patient was diagnosed as having _____. This is a type of kidney disease caused by inflammation of the glomeruli that causes red blood cells and proteins to leak into the urine.

9.75. Mrs. Franklin describes her condition as a floating kidney. The medical term for this condition, in which there is a dropping down of the kidney, is _____.

Which Is the Correct Medical Term?

Select the correct answer, and write it on the line provided.

9.76. Acute renal failure has sudden onset and is characterized by _____. This condition can be caused by many factors, including a sudden drop in blood volume or blood pressure due to injury or surgery.

    anuria   dysuria   enuresis   uremia

9.77. The term _____ means urinary incontinence during sleep. It is also known as bed-wetting.

    nocturnal enuresis   overactive bladder   stress incontinence   urinary incontinence

9.78. The term meaning the distention of the ureter is _____.

    ureteritis   ureterectasis   ureterolith   urethrostenosis

9.79. The presence of abnormally *low* concentrations of protein in the blood is known as _____.

    hyperplasia   hyperproteinuria   hypocalcemia   hypoproteinemia

9.80. A specialist in diagnosing and treating diseases and disorders of the kidneys is a/an _____.

    gynecologist   nephrologist   proctologist   urologist

Challenge Word Building

These terms are *not* found in this chapter; however, they are made up of the following familiar word parts. If you need help in creating the term, refer to your medical dictionary.

cyst/o	**-cele**
nephr/o	**-itis**
pyel/o	**-lysis**
ureter/o	**-malacia**
urethr/o	**-ostomy**
	-otomy
	-plasty
	-ptosis
	-rrhexis
	-sclerosis

9.81. The creation of an artificial opening between the urinary bladder and the exterior of the body is a/an _____.

9.82. A surgical incision into the kidney is a/an _____.

9.83. Abnormal hardening of the kidney is known as _____.

9.84. Prolapse of the bladder into the urethra is known as _____.

9.85. A prolapse of the female urethra is a/an _____.

9.86. The procedure to separate adhesions around a ureter is a/an _____.

9.87. Abnormal softening of the kidney is known as _____.

9.88. Inflammation of the renal pelvis and kidney is known as _____.

9.89. The surgical creation of an outside excretory opening from the urethra is a/an _____.

9.90. The surgical repair of the bladder is a/an _____.

Labeling Exercises

Identify the numbered items on the accompanying figure.

9.91. _____ gland

9.92. exterior view of the right _____

9.93. inferior _____

9.94. _____

9.95. renal _____

9.96. renal _____

9.97. abdominal _____

9.98. right and left _____

9.99. urinary _____

9.100. urethral _____

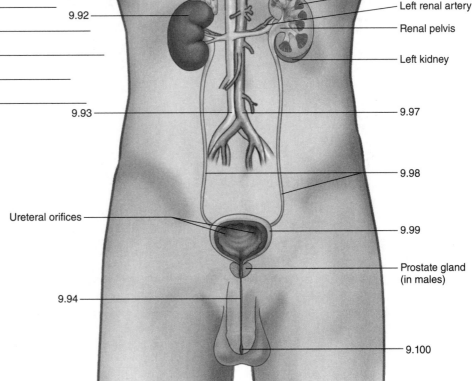

CHAPTER 10

The Nervous System

Learning Exercises

Class _____   Name _____

Matching Word Parts 1

Write the correct answer in the middle column.

Definition	Correct Answer	Possible Answers
10.1. feeling	_____	**psych/o**
10.2. brain	_____	**encephal/o**
10.3. bruise	_____	**contus/o**
10.4. mind	_____	**concuss/o**
10.5. shaken together	_____	**esthet/o**

Matching Word Parts 2

Write the correct answer in the middle column.

Definition	Correct Answer	Possible Answers
10.6. brain covering	_____	**-esthesia**
10.7. process of producing a picture	_____	**-graphy**
10.8. sensation, feeling	_____	**radicul/o**
10.9. spinal cord	_____	**mening/o**
10.10. nerve root	_____	**myel/o**

Matching Word Parts 3

Write the correct answer in the middle column.

Definition	Correct Answer	Possible Answers
10.11. abnormal fear	_____	**-tropic**
10.12. burning sensation	_____	**phobia**
10.13. brain	_____	**neur/o**
10.14. nerve, nerves	_____	**cerebr/o**
10.15. having an affinity for	_____	**caus/o**

Definitions

Select the correct answer, and write it on the line provided.

10.16. The space between two neurons or between a neuron and a receptor organ is known as a
_____.

     dendrite   ganglion   plexus   synapse

10.17. The white protective covering over some parts of the spinal cord and the axon of most peripheral nerves is the _____.

     myelin sheath   neuroglia   neurotransmitter   pia mater

10.18. The _____ are the root-like structures of a nerve that receive impulses and conduct them to the cell body.

     axons   dendrites   ganglions   neurotransmitters

10.19. The _____ is the layer of the meninges that is located nearest to the brain and spinal cord.

     arachnoid membrane   dura mater   meninx   pia mater

10.20. Seven vital body functions are regulated by the _____.

     cerebral cortex   cerebellum   hypothalamus   thalamus

10.21. The _____ nerves are the division of the autonomic nervous system that prepare the body for emergencies and stress.

     afferent   parasympathetic   peripheral   sympathetic

10.22. A _____ is a network of intersecting nerves.

     ganglion   plexus   synapse   tract

10.23. Cranial nerves are part of the _____ nervous system.

     autonomic   central   cranial   peripheral

10.24. The _____ relays sensory stimuli from the spinal cord and midbrain to the cerebral cortex.

     cerebellum   hypothalamus   medulla oblongata   thalamus

10.25. The _____ neurons carry impulses away from the brain and spinal cord.

     afferent   associative   efferent   sensory

Matching Structures

Write the correct answer in the middle column.

Definition	Correct Answer	Possible Answers
10.26. connects the brain and spinal cord	_____	medulla oblongata
10.27. controls vital body functions	_____	hypothalamus
10.28. coordinates muscular activity	_____	cerebrum
10.29. controls basic survival functions	_____	cerebellum
10.30. uppermost layer of the brain	_____	brainstem

Which Word?

Select the correct answer, and write it on the line provided.

10.31. A physician who specializes in administering anesthetic agents is an _____.

anesthetist   anesthesiologist

10.32. A _____ is a profound state of unconsciousness marked by the absence of spontaneous eye movements, no response to painful stimuli, and the lack of speech.

coma   stupor

10.33. An _____ drug is also known as a tranquilizer.

antipsychotic   anxiolytic

10.34. A/An _____ is a sensory perception that has no basis in external stimulation.

delusion   hallucination

10.35. An excessive fear of heights is _____.

acrophobia   agoraphobia

Spelling Counts

Find the misspelled word in each sentence. Then write that word, spelled correctly, on the line provided.

10.36. A migrane headache is characterized by throbbing pain on one side of the head.

_____

10.37. Alzhiemer's disease is a group of disorders involving the parts of the brain that control thought, memory, and language. _____

10.38. An anasthetic is the medication used to induce anesthesia. _____

10.39. Epalepsy is a chronic neurological condition characterized by recurrent episodes of seizures of varying severity. _____

10.40. Siatica is a nerve inflammation that results in pain, burning, and tingling through the thigh, leg, and foot. _____

Abbreviation Identification

In the space provided, write the words that each abbreviation stands for.

10.41. **CP** _____

10.42. **CSF** _____

10.43. **OCD** _____

10.44. **PTSD** _____

10.45. **TIA** _____

Term Selection

Select the correct answer, and write it on the line provided.

10.46. The acute condition that is characterized by confusion, disorientation, disordered thinking and memory, agitation, and hallucinations is known as _____.

    delirium   dementia   lethargy   stupor

10.47. The term meaning inflammation of the spinal cord is _____. This term also means inflammation of bone marrow.

    encephalitis   myelitis   myelosis   radiculitis

10.48. The medical term meaning an abnormal fear of being in small or enclosed spaces is

_____.

    acrophobia   claustrophobia   kleptomania   pyromania

10.49. The condition known as _____ is characterized by severe lightning-like pain due to an inflammation of the fifth cranial nerve.

    Bell's palsy   Guillain-Barré syndrome   Lou Gehrig's disease   trigeminal neuralgia

10.50. The medical term for the condition also known as a developmental reading disorder is

_____.

    autism   dissociative disorder   dyslexia   mental retardation

Sentence Completion

Write the correct term or terms on the lines provided.

10.51. A _____ is the bruising of brain tissue as the result of a head injury.

10.52. The mental conditions characterized by excessive, irrational dread of everyday situations or fear that is out of proportion to the real danger in a situation are known as _____.

10.53. A low-grade chronic depression with symptoms that are milder than those of severe depression but are present on a majority of days for two or more years is known as _____.

10.54. A/An _____ disorder is a condition in which an individual acts as if he or she has a physical or mental illness when he or she is not really sick.

10.55. A/An _____ drug is administered to treat symptoms of severe disorders of thinking and mood that are associated with neurological and psychiatric illnesses such as schizophrenia, mania, and delusional disorders.

Word Surgery

Divide each term into its component word parts. Write these word parts, in sequence, on the lines provided. When necessary, use a slash (/) to indicate a combining vowel. (You may not need all of the lines provided.)

10.56. An **anesthetic** is the medication used to induce anesthesia.

_____   _____   _____   _____

10.57. **Somnambulism** is commonly known as sleepwalking.

_____   _____   _____   _____

10.58. **Electroencephalography** is the process of recording the electrical activity of the brain through the use of electrodes attached to the scalp.

_____   _____   _____   _____

10.59. **Paresthesia** refers to a burning or prickling sensation that is usually felt in the hands, arms, legs, or feet.

_____   _____   _____   _____

10.60. **Poliomyelitis** is a contagious viral infection of the brainstem and spinal cord, which sometimes leads to paralysis.

_____   _____   _____   _____

True/False

If the statement is true, write **True** on the line. If the statement is false, write **False** on the line.

10.61. _____ A hemorrhagic stroke occurs when a blood vessel in the brain leaks.

10.62. _____ An absence seizure is a brief disturbance in brain function in which there is a loss of awareness.

10.63. _____ A sedative is administered to prevent the seizures associated with epilepsy.

10.64. _____ A patient in a persistent vegetative state sleeps through the night and is awake and conscious during the day.

10.65. _____ A psychotropic drug acts primarily on the central nervous system where it produces temporary changes affecting the mind, emotions, and behavior.

Clinical Conditions

Write the correct answer on the line provided.

10.66. Harvey Ikeman has mood shifts from highs to severe lows that affect his attitude, energy, and ability to function. Harvey's doctor describes this condition as a/an _____ disorder.

10.67. In the auto accident, Anthony DeNicola hit his head on the windshield. The paramedics were concerned that this jarring of the brain had caused a/an _____.

10.68. Georgia Houghton suffered a _____ attack (TIA), and her doctors were concerned that this was a warning of an increased stroke risk.

10.69. To control her patient's tremors caused by Parkinson's disease, Dr. Wang performed a/an _____. This is a surgical incision into the thalamus.

10.70. Mary Beth Cawthorn was diagnosed as having _____. This progressive autoimmune disease is characterized by inflammation that causes demyelination of the myelin sheath.

10.71. After several months of being unable to sleep well, Wayne Ladner visited his doctor about this problem. His doctor recorded this condition as being _____.

10.72. After her stroke, Rosita Valladares was unable to understand written or spoken words. This condition is known as _____.

10.73. Jill Beck said she fainted. The medical term for this brief loss of consciousness caused by the decreased blood flow to the brain is _____.

10.74. The Baily baby was born with _____. This condition is an abnormally increased amount of cerebrospinal fluid in the ventricles of the brain.

10.75. The MRI indicated that Mrs. Hoshi had a collection of blood trapped in the tissues of her brain. This condition, which was caused by a head injury, is called a cranial _____.

Which Is the Correct Medical Term?

Select the correct answer, and write it on the line provided.

10.76. Persistent, severe burning pain that usually follows an injury to a sensory nerve is known as
_____.

causalgia   hyperesthesia   hypoesthesia   paresthesia

10.77. The classification of drug that depresses the central nervous system and usually produces sleep is known as a/an _____.

anesthetic   barbiturate   hypnotic   sedative

10.78. A/An _____ disorder is characterized by serious temporary or ongoing changes in function, such as paralysis or blindness, that are triggered by psychological factors rather than by any physical cause.

anxiety   conversion   factitious   panic

10.79. During childbirth, _____ anesthesia is administered to numb the nerves from the uterus and birth passage without stopping labor.

epidural   local   regional   topical

10.80. The condition known as _____ is a rapidly progressive neurological disease that attacks the nerve cells responsible for controlling voluntary muscles.

amyotrophic lateral sclerosis   cerebral palsy   epilepsy   multiple sclerosis

Challenge Word Building

These terms are *not* found in this chapter; however, they are made up of the following familiar word parts. If you need help in creating the term, refer to your medical dictionary.

poly-	encephal/o	-algia
	mening/o	-itis
	myel/o	-malacia
	neur/o	-oma
		-pathy

10.81. Based on word parts, the term meaning inflammation of the nerves and spinal cord is _____.

10.82. Abnormal softening of the meninges is known as _____.

10.83. A benign neoplasm made up of nerve tissue is a/an _____.

10.84. Based on word parts, the term meaning any degenerative disease of the brain is _____.

10.85. Pain affecting many nerves is known as _____.

10.86. Abnormal softening of nerve tissue is known as _____.

10.87. Inflammation of the meninges and the brain is known as _____.

10.88. Based on word parts, the term meaning any pathological condition of the spinal cord is _____.

10.89. Abnormal softening of the brain is known as _____.

10.90. Inflammation of the meninges, brain, and spinal cord is known as _____.

Labeling Exercises

Identify the numbered items on the accompanying figures.

10.91. _____ cortex

10.92. _____ lobe

10.93. _____ lobe

10.94. _____ lobe

10.95. _____ lobe

10.96. _____

10.97. _____

10.98. _____

10.99. _____ cord

10.100. _____

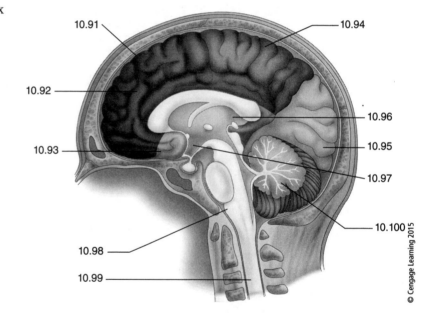

© Cengage Learning 2015

Special Senses: The Eyes and Ears

Learning Exercises

Class _____   Name _____

Matching Word Parts 1

Write the correct answer in the middle column.

Definition	Correct Answer	Possible Answers
11.1. cornea, hard	_____	opt/o
11.2. eyelid	_____	-metry
11.3. eye, vision	_____	kerat/o
11.4. hearing	_____	-cusis
11.5. to measure	_____	blephar/o

Matching Word Parts 2

Write the correct answer in the middle column.

Definition	Correct Answer	Possible Answers
11.6. eardrum	_____	presby/o
11.7. eye, vision	_____	-opia
11.8. iris of the eye	_____	ophthalm/o
11.9. old age	_____	myring/o
11.10. vision condition	_____	irid/o

Matching Word Parts 3

Write the correct answer in the middle column.

Definition	Correct Answer	Possible Answers
11.11. ear	_____	**tympan/o**
11.12. eardrum	_____	**trop/o**
11.13. hard, white of eye	_____	**scler/o**
11.14. retina	_____	**retin/o**
11.15. turn	_____	**ot/o**

Definitions

Select the correct answer, and write it on the line provided.

11.16. The _____ is the structure that maintains the shape of the eye and protects the delicate inner layers of tissue.

| choroid | conjunctiva | cornea | sclera |

11.17. The _____ is the snail-shaped structure of the inner ear.

| cochlea | incus | tarsus | stapes |

11.18. The _____ is also known as the blind spot of the eye.

| fovea centralis | macula | optic disk | optic nerve |

11.19. The _____ lie/s between the outer ear and the middle ear.

| mastoid cells | oval window | posterior segment | tympanic membrane |

11.20. The _____ separates the middle ear from the inner ear.

| eustachian tube | inner canthus | oval window | tympanic membrane |

11.21. The auditory ossicle, which is also known as the anvil, is the _____.

| incus | labyrinth | malleus | stapes |

11.22. The term meaning common changes in the eyes that occur with aging is _____.

| ametropia | amblyopia | presbyopia | presbycusis |

11.23. In _____, a laser is used to repair a detached retina.

| keratoplasty | photocoagulation | retinopexy | trabeculoplasty |

11.24. The turning inward of the edge of the eyelid is known as _____.

| ectropion | emmetropia | entropion | esotropia |

11.25. An inflammation of the middle ear is also called _____.

| mastoiditis | otitis media | infectious myringitis | otalgia |

Matching Conditions

Write the correct answer in the middle column.

Definition	Correct Answer	Possible Answers
11.26. cross-eyes	_____	exotropia
11.27. double vision	_____	myopia
11.28. farsightedness	_____	hyperopia
11.29. nearsightedness	_____	esotropia
11.30. walleye	_____	diplopia

Which Word?

Select the correct answer, and write it on the line provided.

11.31. A _____ is the unit of measurement of a lens's refractive power.

decibel   diopter

11.32. The term meaning bleeding from the ears is _____.

otorrhagia   otorrhea

11.33. A _____ is the surgical incision of the eardrum to create an opening for the placement of ear tubes.

myringotomy   tympanoplasty

11.34. A visual field test to determine losses in peripheral vision is used to diagnose

_____.

cataracts   glaucoma

11.35. An inflammation of the uvea, causing swelling and irritation, is called _____.

corneal abrasion   uveitis

Spelling Counts

Find the misspelled word in each sentence. Then write that word, spelled correctly, on the line provided.

11.36. The eustashian tubes lead from the middle ear to the nasal cavity and the throat.

_____

11.37. Cerunem, also known as earwax, is secreted by glands that line the external auditory canal.

_____

11.38. Astegmatism is a condition in which the eye does not focus properly because of uneven curvatures of the cornea. _____

11.39. Laberinthitis is an inflammation of the labyrinth that can result in vertigo and deafness.

_____

11.40. A Snellan chart is used to measure visual acuity. _____

Abbreviation Identification

In the space provided, write the words that each abbreviation stands for.

11.41. **CI** _____

11.42. **IOL** _____

11.43. **OD** _____

11.44. **IOP** _____

11.45. **MD** _____

Term Selection

Select the correct answer, and write it on the line provided.

11.46. A radial keratotomy is performed to treat _____.

    cataracts   hyperopia   myopia   strabismus

11.47. The condition in which the pupils are unequal in size is known as _____.

    anisocoria   choked disk   macular degeneration   astigmatism

11.48. A _____ is performed in preparation for the placement of a cochlear implant.

    keratoplasty   labyrinthectomy   mastoidectomy   myringoplasty

11.49. The condition also known as a stye is a _____.

    blepharoptosis   chalazion   hordeolum   subconjunctival hemorrhage

11.50. The medical term for a fungal infection of the external auditory canal is

    _____.

    otalgia   otitis   otomycosis   otopyorrhea

Sentence Completion

Write the correct term or terms on the lines provided.

11.51. The ability of the lens to bend light rays so they focus on the retina is known as

    _____.

11.52. A sense of whirling, dizziness, and the loss of balance is called _____.

11.53. A/An _____ is a specialist in measuring the accuracy of vision.

11.54. An inflammation of the cornea that can be due to many causes, including bacterial, viral, or fungal infections, is known as _____.

11.55. The medical term meaning color blindness is _____.

Word Surgery

Divide each term into its component word parts. Write these word parts, in sequence, on the lines provided. When necessary, use a slash (/) to indicate a combining vowel. (You may not need all of the lines provided.)

11.56. **Anisocoria** is a condition in which the pupils are unequal in size.

_____   _____   _____   _____

11.57. **Emmetropia** is the normal relationship between the refractive power of the eye and the shape of the eye that enables light rays to focus correctly on the retina.

_____   _____   _____   _____

11.58. **Otopyorrhea** is the flow of pus from the ear.

_____   _____   _____   _____

11.59. **Presbycusis** is a gradual loss of sensorineural hearing that occurs as the body ages.

_____   _____   _____   _____

11.60. **Xerophthalmia** is drying of eye surfaces, including the conjunctiva, that is often associated with aging.

_____   _____   _____   _____

True/False

If the statement is true, write **True** on the line. If the statement is false, write **False** on the line.

11.61. _____ Rods in the retina are the receptors for color.

11.62. _____ Aqueous humor is drained through the canal of Schlemm.

11.63. _____ Visual field testing is performed to determine the presence of cataracts.

11.64. _____ Dacryoadenitis is an inflammation of the lacrimal gland caused by a bacterial, viral, or fungal infection.

11.65. _____ Tarsorrhaphy is the suturing together of the upper and lower eyelids.

Clinical Conditions

Write the correct answer on the line provided.

11.66. Following a boxing match, Jack Lawson required _____ to repair the injured pinna of his ear.

11.67. During his scuba diving expedition, Jose Ortega suffered from pressure-related ear discomfort. The medical term for this condition is _____.

11.68. Margo Spencer was diagnosed with closed-angle glaucoma affecting her left eye. She is scheduled to have a/an _____ performed to treat this condition.

11.69. Edward Cooke was diagnosed as having _____. This condition is characterized by blindness in one-half of the visual field.

11.70. While gathering branches after the storm, Vern Passman scratched the cornea of his eye. To diagnose the damage, his ophthalmologist performed _____ staining, which caused the corneal abrasions to appear bright green.

11.71. Ted Milligan was treated for an allergic reaction to being stung by a wasp. His reaction was swelling of the tissues around his eyes, and this is known as _____ edema.

11.72. Adrienne Jacobus is unable to drive at night because she suffers from night blindness. The medical term for this condition is _____.

11.73. James Escobar complained of a ringing sound in his ears. His physician refers to this condition as _____.

11.74. The obstruction of a sebaceous gland caused the _____ to form on Ingrid Clareus' upper eyelid.

11.75. Susie Harris was diagnosed as having _____. Her mother referred to this condition as pinkeye.

Which Is the Correct Medical Term?

Select the correct answer, and write it on the line provided.

11.76. Commonly known as choked disk, _____ is swelling and inflammation of the optic nerve at the point of entrance into the eye through the optic disk.

dilation   papilledema   tinnitus   xerophthalmia

11.77. The presence of what appear to be flashes of light is known as _____.

blind spot   retinal detachment   floaters   photopsia

11.78. The term _____ describes any error of refraction in which images do not focus properly on the retina.

ametropia   diplopia   esotropia   hemianopia

11.79. The _____ is the angle where the upper and lower eyelids meet.

canthus   lacrimal glands   conjunctiva   tarsus

11.80. The term _____ describes an accumulation of earwax that forms a solid mass by adhering to the walls of the external auditory canal.

canthus   impacted cerumen   otitis externa   mastoiditis

Challenge Word Building

These terms are *not* found in this chapter; however, they are made up of the following familiar word parts. If you need help in creating the term, refer to your medical dictionary.

blephar/o	**-algia**
irid/o	**-ectomy**
labyrinth/o	**-edema**
lacrim/o	**-itis**
ophthalm/o	**-ology**
retin/o	**-otomy**
	-pathy

11.81. Pain felt in the iris is known as _____.

11.82. Inflammation of the eyelid is known as _____.

11.83. Inflammation of the lacrimal duct is _____.

11.84. Based on word parts, the term _____ means any disease of the eyelid.

11.85. The medical specialty concerned with the eye, its diseases, and refractive errors is known as _____.

11.86. Swelling of the eyelid is known as _____.

11.87. A surgical incision into the lacrimal duct is a/an _____.

11.88. A surgical incision into the labyrinth of the inner ear is a/an _____.

11.89. The term meaning any disease of the iris is _____.

11.90. The surgical removal of the retina is known as a/an _____.

Labeling Exercises

Identify the numbered items on the accompanying figures.

11.91. _____

11.92. anterior _____

11.93. crystalline _____

11.94. _____

11.95. _____ centralis

11.96. _____ or auricle

11.97. external _____ canal

11.98. _____ membrane

11.99. _____ tube

11.100. _____

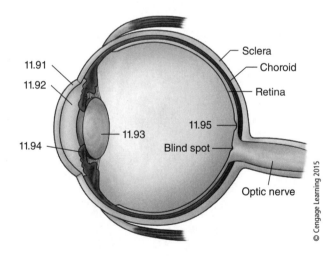

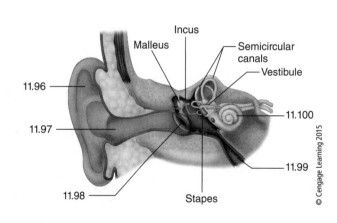

Skin: The Integumentary System

Learning Exercises

Class _____   Name _____

Matching Word Parts 1

Write the correct answer in the middle column.

Definition	Correct Answer	Possible Answers
12.1. skin	_____	**urtic/o**
12.2. rash	_____	**rhytid/o**
12.3. red	_____	**hidr/o**
12.4. sweat	_____	**erythr/o**
12.5. wrinkle	_____	**cutane/o**

Matching Word Parts 2

Write the correct answer in the middle column.

Definition	Correct Answer	Possible Answers
12.6. black, dark	_____	**pedicul/o**
12.7. fat, lipid	_____	**melan/o**
12.8. horny, hard	_____	**lip/o**
12.9. lice	_____	**kerat/o**
12.10. skin	_____	**dermat/o**

Matching Word Parts 3

Write the correct answer in the middle column.

Definition	Correct Answer	Possible Answers
12.11. dry	_____	**xer/o**
12.12. fungus	_____	**seb/o**
12.13. hairy, rough	_____	**onych/o**
12.14. nail	_____	**myc/o**
12.15. sebum	_____	**hirsut/o**

Definitions

Select the correct answer, and write it on the line provided.

12.16. An acute, rapidly spreading bacterial infection within the connective tissues is known as _____

    abscess   cellulitis   fissure   ulcer

12.17. Atypical moles that can develop into skin cancer are known as _____.

    dysplastic nevi   lipomas   malignant keratoses   papillomas

12.18. The autoimmune disorder in which there are well-defined bald areas is known as _____

    alopecia areata   alopecia capitis   alopecia universalis   psoriasis

12.19. A/An _____ is a swelling of clotted blood trapped in the tissues.

    abscess   contusion   hematoma   petechiae

12.20. The term _____ means profuse sweating.

    anhidrosis   diaphoresis   hidrosis   ecchymosis

12.21. A normal scar resulting from the healing of a wound is called a _____.

    cicatrix   keloid   keratosis   papilloma

12.22. A large blister that is usually more than 0.5 cm in diameter is known as a/an _____.

    abscess   bulla   pustule   vesicle

12.23. The removal of dirt, foreign objects, damaged tissue, and cellular debris from a wound is called _____.

    cauterization   curettage   debridement   dermabrasion

12.24. A _____ burn has blisters plus damage only to the epidermis and dermis.

    first-degree   fourth-degree   second-degree   third-degree

12.25. Commonly known as warts, _____ are small, hard skin lesions caused by the human papillomavirus.

    nevi   petechiae   scabies   verrucae

Matching Structures

Write the correct answer in the middle column.

Definition	Correct Answer	Possible Answers
12.26. fibrous protein found in hair, nails, and skin	_____	unguis
12.27. fingernail or toenail	_____	sebaceous glands
12.28. glands secreting sebum	_____	mammary glands
12.29. milk-producing sebaceous glands	_____	keratin
12.30. the layer of tissue below the epidermis	_____	dermis

Which Word?

Select the correct answer, and write it on the line provided.

12.31. The medical term for the condition commonly known as an ingrown toenail is
_____.

    onychomycosis   onychocryptosis

12.32. The bacterial skin infection characterized by isolated pustules that become crusted and rupture is known as _____. This highly contagious condition commonly occurs in children.

    impetigo   xeroderma

12.33. A torn or jagged wound or an accidental cut wound is known as a _____.

    laceration   lesion

12.34. The lesions of _____ carcinoma tend to bleed easily.

    basal cell   squamous cell

12.35. Group A strep, also known as flesh-eating bacteria, causes _____.

    systematic lupus erythematosus   necrotizing fasciitis

Spelling Counts

Find the misspelled word in each sentence. Then write that word, spelled correctly, on the line provided.

12.36. Soriasis is a disease of the skin characterized by itching and by red papules covered with silvery scales. _____

12.37. Exema is an inflammatory skin disease with possible blistering, cracking, oozing, or bleeding. _____

12.38. An absess is a localized collection of pus. _____

12.39. Onichia is an inflammation of the nail bed that usually results in the loss of the nail. _____

12.40. Schleroderma is an autoimmune disorder in which the connective tissues become thickened and hardened, causing the skin to become hard and swollen. _____

Abbreviation Identification

In the space provided, write the words that each abbreviation stands for.

12.41. **BCC** _____

12.42. **I & D** _____

12.43. **SLE** _____

12.44. **MM** _____

12.45. **SCC** _____

Term Selection

Select the correct answer, and write it on the line provided.

12.46. A _____ is a small, knot-like swelling of granulation tissue in the epidermis.

  cicatrix   granuloma   keratosis   petechiae

12.47. An infestation of lice is known as _____

  pediculosis   itch mites   cicatrix   scabies

12.48. The term _____ is used to describe any redness of the skin due to dilated capillaries.

  dermatitis   ecchymosis   erythema   urticaria

12.49. Flakes or dry patches made up of excess dead epidermal cells are known as

_____.

  bullae   macules   plaques   scales

12.50. A cluster of connected boils is known as a/an _____.

  acne vulgaris   carbuncle   comedo   furuncle

Sentence Completion

Write the correct term or terms on the lines provided.

12.51. The term meaning producing or containing pus is _____.

12.52. The term meaning a fungal infection of the nail is _____.

12.53. Tissue death followed by bacterial invasion and putrefaction is known as _____.

12.54. A genetic condition characterized by a deficiency or absence of pigment in the skin, hair, and irises is known as _____.

12.55. Commonly known as hives, _____ are itchy wheals caused by an allergic reaction.

Word Surgery

Divide each term into its component word parts. Write these word parts, in sequence, on the lines provided. When necessary use a slash (/) to indicate a combining vowel. (You may not need all of the lines provided.)

12.56. A **rhytidectomy** is the surgical removal of excess skin for the elimination of wrinkles.

_____ _____ _____ _____

12.57. **Onychomycosis** is a fungal infection of the nail.

_____ _____ _____ _____

12.58. **Folliculitis** is an inflammation of the hair follicles that is especially common on the limbs and in the beard area of men.

_____ _____ _____ _____

12.59. **Pruritus**, which is commonly known as itching, is associated with most forms of dermatitis.

_____ _____ _____ _____

12.60. **Ichthyosis** is a group of hereditary disorders that are characterized by dry, thickened, and scaly skin.

_____ _____ _____ _____

True/False

If the statement is true, write **True** on the line. If the statement is false, write **False** on the line.

12.61. _____ An actinic keratosis is a precancerous skin growth that occurs on sun-damaged skin.

12.62. _____ A skin tag is a malignant skin enlargement commonly found on older clients.

12.63. _____ The arrector pili cause the raised areas of skin known as goose bumps.

12.64. _____ A keratosis is an abnormally raised scar.

12.65. _____ Lipedema, which is also known as painful fat syndrome, affects mostly women.

Clinical Conditions

Write the correct answer on the line provided.

12.66. Carmella Espinoza underwent _____ for the treatment of spider veins.

12.67. Jordan Caswell is an albino. This disorder, which is known as _____, is due to a missing enzyme necessary for the production of melanin.

12.68. Soon after Ying Li hit his thumb with a hammer, a collection of blood formed beneath the nail. This condition is a subungual _____.

12.69. Trisha Bell fell off her bicycle and scraped off the superficial layers of skin on her knees. This type of injury is known as a/an _____.

12.70. Molly Malone had a severe fever, and then she developed very small, pinpoint hemorrhages under her skin. The doctor described these as being _____.

12.71. Many of the children in the Happy Hours Day Care Center required treatment for _____, a skin infection caused by an infestation of itch mites.

12.72. Dr. Liu treated Jeanette Isenberg's skin cancer with _____ surgery. With this technique, individual layers of cancerous tissue are removed and examined under a microscope until all cancerous tissue has been removed.

12.73. Mrs. Garrison had cosmetic surgery that is commonly known as a lid lift. The medical term for this surgical treatment is a/an _____.

12.74. Manuel Fernandez developed a/an _____. This condition is a closed pocket containing pus that is caused by a bacterial infection.

12.75. Agnes Farrington calls them night sweats; however, the medical term for this condition is _____.

Which Is the Correct Medical Term?

Select the correct answer, and write it on the line provided.

12.76. The term that refers to an acute infection of the fold of skin around a nail is _____.

onychia   onychocryptosis   paronychia   vitiligo

12.77. When the sebum plug of a _____ is exposed to air, it oxidizes and becomes a blackhead.

chloasma   comedo   macule   pustule

12.78. The condition known as _____ is a skin disorder characterized by flare-ups of red papules covered with silvery scales.

chloasma   psoriasis   rosacea   eczema

12.79. The medical term referring to a malformation of the nail is _____. This condition is also called spoon nail.

clubbing   koilonychia   onychomycosis   paronychia

12.80. Commonly known as a mole, a/an _____ is a small, dark, skin growth that develops from melanocytes in the skin.

keloid   nevus   papilloma   verrucae

Challenge Word Building

These terms are *not* found in this chapter; however, they are made up of the following familiar word parts. If you need help in creating the term, refer to your medical dictionary.

an-	dermat/o	-derma
hypo-	hidr/o	-ectomy
	melan/o	-ia
	myc/o	-itis
	onych/o	-malacia
	py/o	-oma
	rhin/o	-osis
		-pathy
		-plasty

12.81. Abnormal softening of the nails is known as _____.

12.82. An abnormal condition resulting in the diminished flow of perspiration is known as _____.

12.83. The plastic surgery procedure to change the shape or size of the nose is a/an _____.

12.84. A tumor arising from the nail bed is known as _____.

12.85. The term meaning any disease marked by abnormal pigmentation of the skin is _____.

12.86. The surgical removal of a finger or toenail is a/an _____.

12.87. The term meaning pertaining to the absence of fingernails or toenails is _____.

12.88. The term meaning any disease of the skin is _____.

12.89. Any disease caused by a fungus is _____.

12.90. An excess of melanin present in an area of inflammation of the skin is known as _____.

Labeling Exercises

Identify the numbered items on the accompanying figures.

12.91. _____

12.92. _____

12.93. _____

12.94. _____

12.95. _____

12.96. _____ layer

12.97. _____ layer

12.98. _____ tissue

12.99. _____ gland

12.100. _____ gland

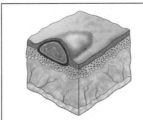

A **12.93** is a small blister containing watery fluid that is less than 0.5 cm in diameter.

© Cengage Learning 2015

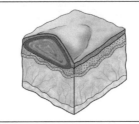

A **12.94** is a large blister that is more than 0.5 cm in diameter.

© Cengage Learning 2015

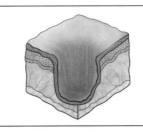

An **12.95** is an open lesion of the skin or mucous membrane, resulting in tissue loss.

© Cengage Learning 2015

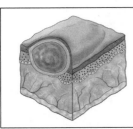

A **12.91** is a closed sack or pouch containing soft or semisolid material.

© Cengage Learning 2015

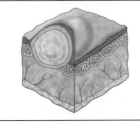

A **12.92** is a small circumscribed elevation of the skin containing pus.

© Cengage Learning 2015

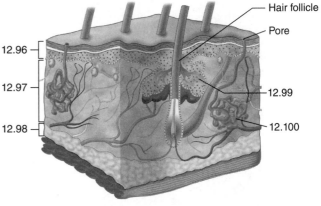

Hair follicle

Pore

12.96

12.97

12.98

12.99

12.100

© Cengage Learning 2015

CHAPTER 13

The Endocrine System

Learning Exercises

Class _____   Name _____

Matching Word Parts 1

Write the correct answer in the middle column.

Definition	Correct Answer	Possible Answers
13.1. adrenal glands	_____	**acr/o**
13.2. extremities	_____	**adren/o**
13.3. ovaries or testicles	_____	**crin/o**
13.4. thirst	_____	**-dipsia**
13.5. to secrete	_____	**gonad/o**

Matching Word Parts 2

Write the correct answer in the middle column.

Definition	Correct Answer	Possible Answers
13.6. condition	_____	**pituitar/o**
13.7. pancreas	_____	**pineal/o**
13.8. parathyroid glands	_____	**parathyroid/o**
13.9. pineal gland	_____	**pancreat/o**
13.10. pituitary gland	_____	**-ism**

Matching Word Parts 3

Write the correct answer in the middle column.

Definition	Correct Answer	Possible Answers
13.11. body	_____	**thym/o**
13.12. many	_____	**thyroid/o**
13.13. sugar	_____	**somat/o**
13.14. thyroid	_____	**poly-**
13.15. thymus	_____	**glyc/o**

Definitions

Select the correct answer, and write it on the line provided.

13.16. The _____ hormone stimulates ovulation in the female.

    estrogen   follicle-stimulating   lactogenic   luteinizing

13.17. The _____ gland secretes hormones that control the activity of the other endocrine glands.

    adrenal   hypothalamus   pituitary   thymus

13.18. The _____ hormone stimulates the growth and secretions of the adrenal cortex.

    adrenocorticotropic   growth   melanocyte-stimulating   thyroid-stimulating

13.19. The _____ gland functions as part of the endocrine system by secreting a hormone that functions as part of the immune system.

    adrenal   parathyroid   pineal   thymus

13.20. The hormone _____ works with the parathyroid hormone to decrease calcium levels in the blood and tissues.

    aldosterone   calcitonin   glucagon   leptin

13.21. Cortisol is secreted by the _____.

    adrenal cortex   adrenal medulla   pituitary gland   thyroid gland

13.22. The amount of glucose in the bloodstream is increased by the hormone _____.

    adrenaline   glucagon   hydrocortisone   insulin

13.23. Norepinephrine is secreted by the _____.

    adrenal cortex   adrenal medulla   pancreatic islets   pituitary gland

13.24. The hormone _____ stimulates uterine contractions during childbirth.

    estrogen   oxytocin   progesterone   testosterone

13.25. The development of the male secondary sex characteristics is stimulated by the hormone _____.

    parathyroid   pitocin   progesterone   testosterone

Matching Structures

Write the correct answer in the middle column.

Definition	Correct Answer	Possible Answers
13.26. controls blood sugar levels	_____	thyroid gland
13.27. controls the activity of other endocrine glands	_____	pituitary gland
13.28. influences the sleep-wakefulness cycle	_____	pineal gland
13.29. regulates electrolyte levels	_____	pancreatic islets
13.30. stimulates metabolism	_____	adrenal glands

Which Word?

Select the correct answer, and write it on the line provided.

13.31. The hormonal disorder that results from too much growth hormone in adults is known as _____.

   acromegaly   gigantism

13.32. The growth hormone is secreted by the _____ of the pituitary gland.

   anterior lobe   posterior lobe

13.33. Diabetes type 2 is an _____ disorder.

   insulin deficiency   insulin resistance

13.34. Insufficient production of ADH causes _____.

   diabetes insipidus   Graves' disease

13.35. _____ is caused by prolonged exposure to high levels of cortisol.

   Addison's disease   Cushing's syndrome

Spelling Counts

Find the misspelled word in each sentence. Then write that word, spelled correctly, on the line provided.

13.36. The lutinizing hormone stimulates ovulation in the female. _____

13.37. Diabetes mellitas is a group of diseases characterized by defects in insulin secretion, insulin action, or both. _____

13.38. Myxedemia is also known as adult hypothyroidism. _____

13.39. The hormone progestarone is released during the second half of the menstrual cycle. _____

13.40. Thymoxin is secreted by the thymus gland. _____

Abbreviation Identification

In the space provided, write the words that each abbreviation stands for.

13.41. **ACTH** _____

13.42. **ADH** _____

13.43. **DM** _____

13.44. **FBS** _____

13.45. **FSH** _____

Term Selection

Select the correct answer, and write it on the line provided.

13.46. A rare life-threatening condition caused by exaggerated hyperthyroidism is called
_____.

      thyroid nodules   goiter   thyroid storm   Graves' disease

13.47. The condition known as _____ is characterized by abnormally high concentrations of calcium circulating in the blood instead of being stored in the bones.

      hypercalcemia   hyperthyroidism   hypocalcemia   polyphagia

13.48. The four _____ glands, each of which is about the size of a grain of rice, are embedded in the posterior surface of the thyroid gland.

      adrenal   pancreatic   parathyroid   pineal

13.49. A/An _____ is a benign tumor of the pituitary gland that causes it to produce too much prolactin.

      insuloma   pheochromocytoma   pituitary adenoma   prolactinoma

13.50. The average blood glucose levels over the past 3 weeks is measured by the
_____ test.

      blood sugar monitoring   fructosamine   glucose tolerance   hemoglobin A1c

Sentence Completion

Write the correct term or terms on the lines provided.

13.51. The mineral substances known as _____ are found in the blood and include sodium and potassium.

13.52. The two primary hormones secreted by the thyroid gland are triiodothyronine (T_3) and _____ (T_4).

13.53. Damage to the retina of the eye caused by diabetes mellitus is known as diabetic
_____.

13.54. The medical term meaning excessive hunger is _____.

13.55. Abnormal protrusion of the eye out of the orbit is known as _____.

Word Surgery

Divide each term into its component word parts. Write these word parts, in sequence, on the lines provided. When necessary, use a slash (/) to indicate a combining vowel. (You may not need all of the lines provided.)

13.56. **Hyperpituitarism** is the excess secretion of growth hormone by the pituitary gland, causing acromegaly and gigantism.

_____ _____ _____ _____

13.57. **Hypoglycemia** is an abnormally low concentration of glucose in the blood.

_____ _____ _____ _____

13.58. **Hyperinsulinism** is the condition of excessive secretion of insulin in the bloodstream.

_____ _____ _____ _____

13.59. **Gynecomastia** is the condition of excessive mammary development in the male.

_____ _____ _____ _____

13.60. **Hypocalcemia** is characterized by abnormally low levels of calcium in the blood.

_____ _____ _____ _____

True/False

If the statement is true, write **True** on the line. If the statement is false, write **False** on the line.

13.61. _____ The beta cells of the pancreatic islets secrete glucagon in response to low blood sugar levels.

13.62. _____ A pheochromocytoma is a rare, benign tumor of the adrenal gland that causes too much release of epinephrine and norepinephrine.

13.63. _____ The hormone melatonin is secreted by the adrenal cortex.

13.64. _____ An insulinoma is a malignant tumor of the pancreas that causes hypoglycemia by secreting insulin.

13.65. _____ Polyuria is excessive urination.

Clinical Conditions

Write the correct answer on the line provided.

13.66. During his nursing studies, Rodney Milne learned that the _____ hormone helps control blood pressure by reducing the amount of water that is excreted through the kidneys.

13.67. Eduardo Chavez complained of being thirsty all the time. His doctor noted this excessive thirst on his chart as _____.

13.68. Mrs. Wei's symptoms included chronic, worsening fatigue, muscle weakness, loss of appetite, and weight loss because her adrenal glands do not produce enough cortisol. Her doctor diagnosed this condition as _____.

13.69. Linda Thomas was diagnosed as having a/an _____. This is a benign tumor of the pancreas that causes hypoglycemia by secreting insulin.

13.70. Patrick Edward has the autoimmune disorder known as _____ in which the body's own antibodies attack and destroy the cells of the thyroid gland.

13.71. Because Joe Dean's ultimate goal was to swim in the Olympics, he was tempted to make illegal use of _____ steroids to increase his strength and muscle mass.

13.72. Holly Yates was surprised to learn that _____, which is a hormone secreted by fat cells, travels to the brain and controls the balance of food intake and energy expenditure.

13.73. As a result of a congenital lack of thyroid secretion, the Vaugh-Eames child suffers from _____, which is a condition of arrested physical and mental development.

13.74. Ray Grovenor is excessively tall and large. This condition, which was caused by excessive secretion of growth hormone before puberty, is known as _____.

13.75. Rosita DeAngelis required the surgical removal of her pancreas. The medical term for this procedure is a/an _____.

Which Is the Correct Medical Term?

Select the correct answer, and write it on the line provided.

13.76. Hormones called _____ are produced and released by neurons in the brain, rather than by the endocrine glands, and delivered to organs and tissues through the bloodstream.

    hormones   neurohormones   neurotransmitters   steroids

13.77. A/An _____ is a slow-growing, benign tumor of the pituitary gland that is a functioning tumor (secreting hormones) or a nonfunctioning tumor (not secreting hormones).

    hyperpituitarism   hypophysectomy   pituitary adenoma   prolactinoma

13.78. _____ disease, which is an autoimmune disorder caused by hyperthyroidism, is often characterized by goiter, exophthalmos, or both.

    Addison's   Cushing's   Graves'   Hashimoto's

13.79. The diabetic emergency caused by very high blood sugar is a/an _____.

    diabetic coma   hypoglycemia   insulin shock   insuloma

13.80. The hormone _____, which is secreted by the pineal gland, influences the sleep-wakefulness cycles.

    glucagon   melatonin   parathyroid   thymosin

Challenge Word Building

These terms are *not* found in this chapter; however, they are made up of the following familiar word parts. If you need help in creating the term, refer to your medical dictionary.

endo-	**adren/o**	**-emia**
	crin/o	**-itis**
	hyper-	**-megaly**
	insulin/o	**-ology**
	pancreat/o	**-oma**
	pineal/o	**-otomy**
	thym/o	**-pathy**
	thyroid/o	

13.81. The term meaning any disease of the adrenal glands is _____.

13.82. The study of endocrine glands and their secretions is known as _____.

13.83. Abnormal enlargement of the adrenal glands is known as _____.

13.84. The term meaning any disease of the thymus gland is _____.

13.85. Inflammation of the thyroid gland is known as _____.

13.86. A surgical incision into the pancreas is a/an _____.

13.87. A surgical incision into the thyroid gland is a/an _____.

13.88. The term meaning any disease of the pineal gland is _____.

13.89. Abnormally high levels of insulin in the blood are known as _____.

13.90. Inflammation of the adrenal glands is known as _____.

Labeling Exercises

Identify the numbered items on the accompanying figure.

13.91. _____ gland

13.92. _____ glands

13.93. _____ gland

13.94. _____ of the female

13.95. _____

13.96. _____ gland

13.97. _____ gland

13.98. _____ glands

13.99. _____ islets

13.100. _____ of the male

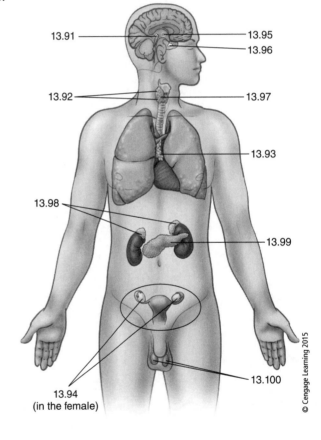

CHAPTER 14

The Reproductive Systems

Learning Exercises

Class _____   Name _____

Matching Word Parts 1

Write the correct answer in the middle column.

Definition	Correct Answer	Possible Answers
14.1. cervix	_____	**men/o**
14.2. female	_____	**gynec/o**
14.3. menstruation	_____	**-gravida**
14.4. pregnant	_____	**colp/o**
14.5. vagina	_____	**cervic/o**

Matching Word Parts 2

Write the correct answer in the middle column.

Definition	Correct Answer	Possible Answers
14.6. egg	_____	**vagin/o**
14.7. ovary	_____	**test/i**
14.8. testicle	_____	**ov/o**
14.9. uterus	_____	**ovari/o**
14.10. vagina	_____	**hyster/o**

Matching Word Parts 3

Write the correct answer in the middle column.

Definition	Correct Answer	Possible Answers
14.11. breast	_____	**salping/o**
14.12. none	_____	**-pexy**
14.13. surgical fixation	_____	**-para**
14.14. to give birth	_____	**nulli-**
14.15. tube	_____	**mast/o**

Definitions

Select the correct answer, and write it on the line provided.

14.16. The term that describes the inner layer of the uterus is _____.

   corpus   endometrium   myometrium   perimetrium

14.17. The term describing the single cells formed immediately after conception is _____.

   embryo   fetus   gamete   zygote

14.18. The mucus that lubricates the vagina is produced by the _____.

   Bartholin's glands   bulbourethral glands   Cowper's glands   hymen glands

14.19. The finger-like structures of the fallopian tube that catch the ovum are the _____.

   fimbriae   fundus   infundibulum   oviducts

14.20. The term _____ is used to designate the transition phase between regular menstrual periods and no periods at all.

   menarche   menopause   perimenopause   puberty

14.21. The medical term for the condition also known as a yeast infection is _____.

   colporrhea   leukorrhea   pruritus vulvae   vaginal candidiasis

14.22. Sperm are formed within the _____ of each testicle.

   ejaculatory ducts   epididymis   seminiferous tubules   urethra

14.23. During puberty, the term _____ describes the beginning of the menstrual function.

   menarche   menopause   menses   menstruation

14.24. In the female, the region between the vaginal orifice and the anus is known as the _____.

   clitoris   mons pubis   perineum   vulva

14.25. The release of a mature egg by the ovary is known as _____.

   coitus   fertilization   menstruation   ovulation

Matching Structures

Write the correct answer in the middle column.

Definition	Correct Answer	Possible Answers
14.26. carry milk from the mammary glands	_____	vulva
14.27. surrounds the testicles	_____	scrotum
14.28. external female genitalia	_____	lactiferous ducts
14.29. protects the tip of the penis	_____	foreskin
14.30. sensitive tissue near the vaginal opening	_____	clitoris

Which Word?

Select the correct answer, and write it on the line provided.

14.31. The term used to describe a woman during her first pregnancy is a _____.

primigravida   primipara

14.32. The fluid produced by the mammary glands during the first few days after giving birth is _____.

colostrum   meconium

14.33. The term _____ describes an inflammation of the cervix that is usually caused by an infection.

cervicitis   vulvitis

14.34. From implantation through the 8th week of pregnancy, the developing child is known as a/an _____.

embryo   fetus

14.35. A _____ is a woman who has never borne a viable child.

nulligravida   nullipara

Spelling Counts

Find the misspelled word in each sentence. Then write that word, spelled correctly, on the line provided.

14.36. The prostrate gland secretes a thick fluid that aids the motility of the sperm.
_____

14.37. The normal periodic discharge from the uterus is known as menstration. _____

14.38. The third stage of labor and delivery is the expulsion of the plasenta as the afterbirth.
_____

14.39. The term hemataspermia is the presence of blood in the seminal fluid. _____

14.40. The surgical removal of the foreskin of the penis is known as cercumsion.
_____

Abbreviation Identification

In the space provided, write the words that each abbreviation stands for.

14.41. **AMA** _____

14.42. **PID** _____

14.43. **PMDD** _____

14.44. **IUD** _____

14.45. **VD** _____

Term Selection

Select the correct answer, and write it on the line provided.

14.46. An accumulation of pus in the fallopian tube is known as _____.

oophoritis   pelvic inflammatory disease   pyosalpinx   salpingitis

14.47. A _____ is a knot of widening varicose veins in one side of the scrotum.

hydrocele   phimosis   priapism   varicocele

14.48. The direct visual examination of the tissues of the cervix and vagina using a binocular magnifier is known as _____.

colposcopy   endovaginal ultrasound   hysteroscopy   laparoscopy

14.49. The term used to describe infrequent or very light menstruation in a woman with previously normal periods is _____.

amenorrhea   hypomenorrhea   oligomenorrhea   polymenorrhea

14.50. The examination of cells retrieved from the edge of the placenta between the 8th and 10th weeks of pregnancy is known as _____.

amniocentesis   chorionic villus sampling   fetal monitoring   pelvimetry

Sentence Completion

Write the correct term or terms on the lines provided.

14.51. The dark-pigmented area surrounding the nipple is known as the _____.

14.52. A fluid-filled sac in the scrotum along the spermatic cord leading from the testicles is known as a/an _____.

14.53. The serious complication of pregnancy that is characterized by convulsions and sometimes coma is known as _____. The treatment for this condition is delivery of the fetus.

14.54. Surgical suturing of a tear in the vagina is known as _____.

14.55. The _____ is the tube that carries blood, oxygen, and nutrients from the placenta to the developing child.

Word Surgery

Divide each term into its component word parts. Write these word parts, in sequence, on the lines provided. When necessary use a slash (/) to indicate a combining vowel. (You may not need all of the lines provided.)

14.56. **Endocervicitis** is an inflammation of the mucous membrane lining of the cervix.

_____ _____ _____ _____

14.57. **Menometrorrhagia** is excessive uterine bleeding at both the usual time of menstrual periods and at other irregular intervals.

_____ _____ _____ _____

14.58. **Hysterosalpingography** is a radiographic examination of the uterus and fallopian tubes.

_____ _____ _____ _____

14.59. **Galactorrhea** is the production of breast milk in a woman who is not breastfeeding.

_____ _____ _____ _____

14.60. **Azoospermia** is the absence of sperm in the semen.

_____ _____ _____ _____

True/False

If the statement is true, write **True** on the line. If the statement is false, write **False** on the line.

14.61. _____ Peyronie's disease causes a sexual dysfunction in which the penis is bent or curved during erection.

14.62. _____ Braxton Hicks contractions are the first true labor pains.

14.63. _____ An Apgar score is an evaluation of a newborn infant's physical status at 1 and 5 minutes after birth.

14.64. _____ Breast augmentation is mammoplasty that is performed to reduce breast size.

14.65. _____ An ectopic pregnancy is a potentially dangerous condition in which a fertilized egg is implanted and begins to develop outside of the uterus.

Clinical Conditions

Write the correct answer on the line provided.

14.66. Baby Ortega was born with cryptorchidism. When this testicle had not descended by the time he was 9 months old, a/an _____ was performed.

14.67. When she went into labor with her first child, Mrs. Hoshi's baby was in a breech presentation. Because of risks associated with this, her obstetrician delivered the baby surgically by performing a/an _____.

14.68. Dawn Grossman was diagnosed as having uterine fibroids that required surgical removal. Her gynecologist scheduled Dawn for a/an _____.

14.69. Rita Chen, who is 25 years old and knows that she is not pregnant, is concerned because she has not had a menstrual period for 3 months. Her doctor described this condition as _____.

14.70. Enrico Flores's physician removed a portion of each vas deferens. The medical term for this sterilization procedure is a/an _____.

14.71. Tiffany Thomas developed a thin, frothy, yellow-green, foul-smelling vaginal discharge. She was diagnosed as having _____, which is caused by the parasite *Trichomonas vaginalis*.

14.72. Mr. Wolford, who is age 65, has been reading a lot about the decrease of testosterone in older men. His physician told him that the medical term for this condition is _____.

14.73. Just before the delivery of her baby, Barbara Klein's obstetrician performed a/an _____ to prevent tearing of the tissues.

14.74. Jane Marsall's pregnancy was complicated by the abnormal implantation of the placenta in the lower portion of the uterus. The medical term for this condition is _____.

14.75. Immediately after birth, the Reicher baby was described as being a newborn or a/an _____.

Which Is the Correct Medical Term?

Select the correct answer, and write it on the line provided.

14.76. The postpartum vaginal discharge during the first several weeks after childbirth is known as _____.

colostrum   involution   lochia   meconium

14.77. Abdominal pain caused by uterine cramps during a menstrual period is known as _____.

dysmenorrhea   hypermenorrhea   menometrorrhagia   polymenorrhea

14.78. The term that describes an inflammation of the glans penis is _____.

phimosis   balanitis   epididymitis   testitis

14.79. An inflammation of the lining of the vagina is known as _____. The most common causes of this condition are bacterial vaginosis, trichomoniasis, and vaginal candidiasis.

cervical dysplasia   cervicitis   colporrhexis   vaginitis

14.80. The term that describes a profuse whitish mucus discharge from the uterus and vagina is _____. This type of discharge can be due to an infection, malignancy, or hormonal changes.

endocervicitis   leukorrhea   pruritus vulvae   vaginitis

Challenge Word Building

These terms are *not* found in this chapter; however, they are made up of the following familiar word parts. If you need help in creating the term, refer to your medical dictionary.

endo-	**hyster/o**	**-cele**
	mast/o	**-dynia**
	metr/i	**-itis**
	oophor/o	**-pexy**
	orchid/o	**-plasty**
	vagin/o	**-rrhaphy**
	vulv/o	**-rrhexis**

14.81. The term meaning a hernia protruding into the vagina is _____.

14.82. The term meaning the surgical repair of one or both testicles is _____.

14.83. The term meaning an inflammation of the endometrium is _____.

14.84. The term meaning the surgical repair of an ovary is a/an _____.

14.85. The term meaning pain in the vagina is _____.

14.86. The term meaning the surgical suturing of the uterus is _____.

14.87. The term meaning a hernia of the uterus, particularly during pregnancy, is a/an
_____.

14.88. The term meaning the surgical fixation of a displaced ovary is _____.

14.89. The term meaning the rupture of the uterus, particularly during pregnancy, is
_____.

14.90. The term meaning an inflammation of the vulva and the vagina is _____.

Labeling Exercises

Identify the numbered items on these accompanying figures.

14.91. _____ bladder

14.92. _____ gland

14.93. _____

14.94. _____

14.95. _____

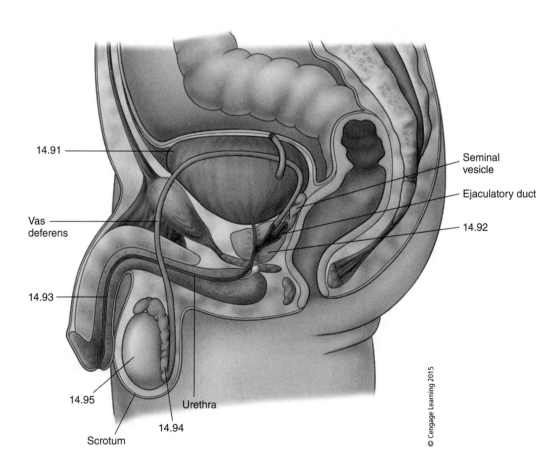

14.96. _____ or uterine tube

14.97. body of the _____

14.98 _____ bladder

14.99. _____

14.100. _____

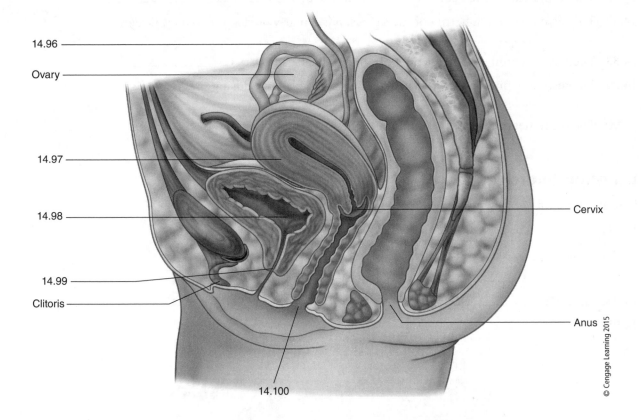

Diagnostic Procedures, Nuclear Medicine, and Pharmacology

Learning Exercises

Class _____   Name _____

Matching Word Parts 1

Write the correct answer in the middle column.

Definition	Correct Answer	Possible Answers
15.1. abdomen	_____	**lapar/o**
15.2. albumin, protein	_____	**glycos/o**
15.3. calcium	_____	**creatin/o**
15.4. creatinine	_____	**calc/i**
15.5. sugar	_____	**albumin/o**

Matching Word Parts 2

Write the correct answer in the middle column.

Definition	Correct Answer	Possible Answers
15.6. surgical puncture to remove fluid	_____	**son/o**
15.7. blood	_____	**-otomy**
15.8. surgical incision	_____	**hemat/o**
15.9. process of producing a picture or record	_____	**-graphy**
15.10. sound	_____	**-centesis**

Matching Word Parts 3

Write the correct answer in the middle column.

Definition	Correct Answer	Possible Answers
15.11. direct visual examination	———————————	**-uria**
15.12. radiation	———————————	**-scopy**
15.13. urine	———————————	**-scope**
15.14. vein	———————————	**radi/o**
15.15. visual examination instrument	———————————	**phleb/o**

Definitions

Select the correct answer, and write it on the line provided.

15.16. The type of therapy in which a patient is placed in a state of focused concentration and narrowed attention that makes him or her more susceptible to suggestions, and then given suggestions directed toward the treatment goal is called ————————————.

mindfulness meditation   hypnosis   biofeedback   guided imagery

15.17. A/An ———————————— is used to enlarge the opening of any body canal or cavity to facilitate inspection of its interior.

endoscope   otoscope   speculum   sphygmomanometer

15.18. The imaging technique that produces multiple cross-sectional images using x-radiation is ————————————.

computed tomography   fluoroscopy   magnetic resonance imaging radiography

15.19. Drug ———————————— is when the body has become accustomed to a medication after being on it for a length of time, and higher doses are required to achieve the desired effect.

tolerance   compliance   side effect   paradoxical reaction

15.20. The diagnostic technique ———————————— creates images of deep body structures by recording the echoes of pulses of sound waves that are above the range of human hearing.

cineradiography   extraoral radiography fluoroscopy   ultrasonography

15.21. The presence of calcium in the urine is known as ————————————.

albuminuria   calciuria   creatinuria   glycosuria

15.22. A/An ———————————— test is used to identify high levels of inflammation within the body.

blood urea nitrogen   C-reactive protein   erythrocyte sedimentation   serum bilirubin

15.23. In the ———————————— position, the patient is lying on the back with the knees bent.

dorsal recumbent   horizontal recumbent knee-chest   supine

15.24. A ———————————— is an abnormal sound heard during auscultation of an artery.

bruit   rale   rhonchi   stridor

15.25. The presence of pus in the urine, which causes the urine to be cloudy or smoky in appearance, is called ————————————.

glycosuria   ketonuria   hematuria   pyuria

Matching Techniques

Write the correct answer in the middle column.

Definition	Correct Answer	Possible Answers
15.26. produces cross-sectional views	———————————————	x-rays
15.27. produces views in only one direction	———————————————	MRI
15.28. the removal of fluid for diagnostic purposes	———————————————	fluoroscopy
15.29. uses a luminous fluorescent screen	———————————————	centesis
15.30. uses radio waves and a magnetic field	———————————————	CT

Which Word?

Select the correct answer, and write it on the line provided.

15.31. A/An _____ reaction is an unexpected reaction to a drug that is peculiar to the individual.

    idiosyncratic   palliative

15.32. _____ tomography combines tomography with radionuclide tracers to produce enhanced images of selected body organs or areas.

    positron emission   single photon emission computed

15.33. A substance that does not allow x-rays to pass through is described as being _____.

    radiolucent   radiopaque

15.34. When film is placed within the mouth and exposed by a camera positioned next to the cheek, this is called _____ radiography.

    extraoral   intraoral

15.35. A _____ drug is sold under the name given to the drug by the manufacturer. These drug names are always spelled with a capital letter.

    brand-name   generic

Spelling Counts

Find the misspelled word in each sentence. Then write that word, spelled correctly, on the line provided.

15.36. Listening through a stethoscope for sounds within the body to determine the condition of the lungs, pleura, heart, and abdomen is known as asultation. _____

15.37. A sphygnomanometer is used to measure blood pressure. _____

15.38. Fluroscopy is the visualization of body parts in motion by projecting x-ray images on a luminous fluorescent screen. _____

15.39. A conterindication is a factor in the patient's condition that makes the use of a medication or specific treatment dangerous or ill advised. _____

15.40. An opthalmoscope is used to examine the interior of the eye. _____

Abbreviation Identification

In the space provided, write the words in English that each abbreviation stands for.

15.41. **ESR** _____

15.42. **NPO** _____

15.43. **prn** _____

15.44. **TPR** _____

15.45. **WBC** _____

Term Selection

Select the correct answer, and write it on the line provided.

15.46. Drawing fluid from the sac surrounding the heart is known as _____.

   abdominocentesis   cardiocentesis   pericardiocentesis   arthrocentesis

15.47. The presence of blood in the urine is known as _____.

   albuminuria   creatinuria   hematuria   ketonuria

15.48. _____ is a combination of nutrition, medicinal supplements and herbs, water therapy, homeopathy, and lifestyle modifications used to identify and treat the root causes of symptoms and disease.

   naturopathy   homeopathy   Qi Gong   biofeedback

15.49. A/An _____ relieves inflammation and pain without affecting consciousness.

   acetaminophen   analgesic   anti-inflammatory   palliative

15.50. The term _____ means the administration of a medication by a manner other than through the digestive tract (more commonly through injection).

   hypodermic   parenteral   transcutaneous   transdermal

Sentence Completion

Write the correct term or terms on the lines provided.

15.51. The term *radiographic* _____ describes the path that the x-ray beam follows through the body from entrance to exit.

15.52. The term _____ describes an abnormal, high-pitched, musical breathing sound that is heard during inspiration.

15.53. A/An _____ is a medical professional trained to draw blood from patients for laboratory tests and other procedures.

15.54. A/An _____ is an instrument used to visually examine the external ear and tympanic membrane.

15.55. _____ is a traditional Chinese touch therapy involving finger pressure applied to specific areas of the body to restore the flow of qi.

Word Surgery

Divide each term into its component word parts. Write these word parts, in sequence, on the lines provided. When necessary use a slash (/) to indicate a combining vowel. (You may not need all of the lines provided.)

15.56. **Arthrocentesis** is a surgical puncture of the joint space to remove synovial fluid for analysis to determine the cause of pain or swelling in a joint.

_____   _____   _____   _____

15.57. **Cineradiography** is the recording of fluoroscopy images.

_____   _____   _____   _____

15.58. **Echocardiography** is an ultrasonic diagnostic procedure used to evaluate the structures and motion of the heart.

_____   _____   _____   _____

15.59. **Bacteriuria** is the presence of bacteria in the urine.

_____   _____   _____   _____

15.60. **Pharmacology** is the study of the nature, uses, and effects of drugs for medical purposes.

_____   _____   _____   _____

True/False

If the statement is true, write **True** on the line. If the statement is false, write **False** on the line.

15.61. _____ Neuromuscular therapy is a form of massage that uses soft-tissue manipulation focusing on applying pressure to trigger points.

15.62. _____ Casts are fibrous or protein materials, such as pus and fats, that are thrown off into the urine in kidney disease.

15.63. _____ A placebo contains medication and has the potential to cure a disease.

15.64. _____ An MRI creates images by combining sound wave pulses and strong magnets.

15.65. _____ Compliance means that the patient has accurately followed instructions.

Clinical Conditions

Write the correct answer on the line provided.

15.66. The urinalysis for Sophia O'Keefe showed the presence of ketones. The medical term for this condition is _____.

15.67. Dr. Jamison suspected her patient had an infection. An elevated count in the patient's _____ cell count test would confirm her diagnosis.

15.68. Kelly Harrison was extremely cold after being stranded in a snowstorm. When rescued, the paramedics said she was suffering from _____.

15.69. During his examination of the patient, Dr. Wong used _____ to feel the texture, size, consistency, and location of certain body parts.

15.70. Dr. McDowell ordered a blood transfusion. Before the transfusion, _____ tests were required to determine the compatibility of donor's and recipient's blood.

15.71. In preparation for his upper GI series, Dwight Oshone swallowed a liquid containing the contrast medium _____.

15.72. Maria Martinez required _____ echocardiography to evaluate the structures of her heart.

15.73. Another term for conventional, or Western, medical practices is _____.

15.74. The urinalysis for Kathleen McCaffee showed _____. This is the presence of glucose in the urine.

15.75. Dr. Roberts used _____ during the examination. This technique involves tapping the surface of the body with a finger or instrument.

Which Is the Correct Medical Term?

Select the correct answer, and write it on the line provided.

15.76. A/An _____ drug reaction is an undesirable reaction that accompanies the principal response for which the drug was taken.

adverse   idiosyncratic   placebo   synergism

15.77. The urinalysis indicated _____. This is an increased concentration of creatinine in the urine.

creatinuria   glycosuria   ketonuria   proteinuria

15.78. The energy therapy where finger pressure is applied to specific areas of the body is called

_____.

Qi Gong   acupuncture   acupressure   hypnosis

15.79. During a/an _____ examination, some patients feel uncomfortable because of the noise generated by the machine and the feeling of being closed in.

CT   MRI   PET   x-ray

15.80. The examination position that has the patient lying on the back with the feet and legs raised and supported in stirrups is the _____ position.

dorsal recumbent   lithotomy   prone   Sims'

Challenge Word Building

These terms are *not* found in this chapter; however, they are made up of the following familiar word parts. If you need help in creating the term, refer to your medical dictionary.

hyper-	**albumin/o**	**-centesis**
hypo-	**calc/i**	**-emia**
	cyst/o	**-gram**
	glycos/o	**-scope**
	protein/o	**-uria**
	pleur/o	
	py/o	

15.81. The term meaning the presence of abnormally low concentrations of protein in the blood is _____.

15.82. The term meaning abnormally high levels of albumin in the blood is _____.

15.83. The term meaning unusually large amounts of sugar in the urine is _____.

15.84. The instrument used to visually examine the interior of the urinary bladder is a/an _____.

15.85. The term meaning a surgical puncture of the chest wall with a needle to obtain fluid from the pleural cavity is _____. This procedure is also known as thoracentesis.

15.86. An x-ray examination of the bladder is called a _____.

15.87. The term meaning an abnormally low level of calcium in the circulating blood is _____.

15.88. The term meaning abnormally large amounts of calcium in the urine is _____.

15.89. The term meaning the presence of pus-forming organisms in the blood is _____.

15.90. The term meaning the presence of excess protein in the urine is _____.

Labeling Exercises

Identify the numbered items on the accompanying figures.

15.91. This is the _____ position.

15.92. This is the _____ recumbent position.

15.93. This is the _____ position.

15.94. This is the _____ recumbent position.

15.95. This is the _____ position.

15.96. This is the _____ position.

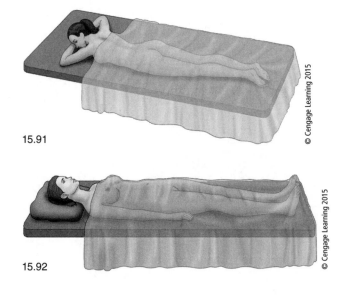

15.91

15.92

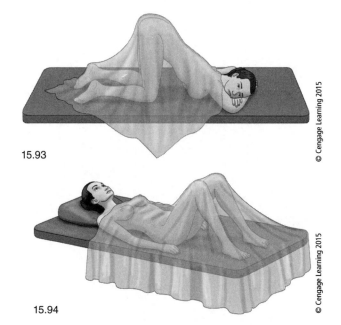

15.93

15.94

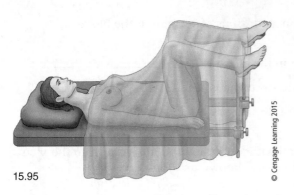

15.95

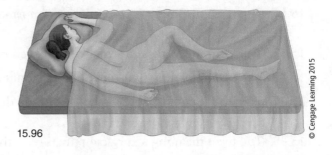

15.96

15.97. This is a/an _____ injection.

15.98. This is a/an _____ injection.

15.99. This is a/an _____ injection.

15.100. This is a/an _____ injection.

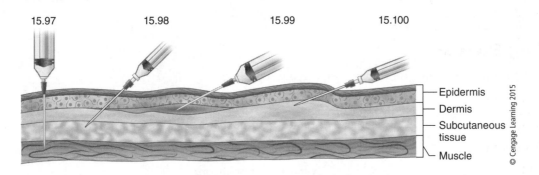

COMPREHENSIVE MEDICAL TERMINOLOGY REVIEW

OVERVIEW OF COMPREHENSIVE MEDICAL TERMINOLOGY REVIEW

Study Tips   Hints to help you review more effectively.

Answer Sheets   Write the *letter* of the correct answer for the questions in the review tests. Although only one set of answer sheets are included, you can take these tests as often as you want.

Review Session   A 100-multiple-choice-question review session to help you determine where you need more study emphasis. However, be aware that none of these questions are from the actual final test.

Simulated Medical   A 100-multiple-choice-question "mock" final test to help you evaluate your progress.
Terminology Final Test   However, be aware that none of these questions are from the actual final test.

STUDY TIPS

Use Your Vocabulary Lists

- Photocopy the vocabulary list for each chapter from your textbook, and add any terms suggested by your instructor. This creates a study aid that is easy to carry with you for additional review whenever you have a free minute.

- Review the terms on each list. When you have mastered a term, put a check in the box next to it. If you cannot spell and define a term, highlight it for further study.

- Look up the meanings of the highlighted terms in the textbook, and work on mastering them.

- When using a list is not convenient, consider listening to the **Audio CDs** that accompany this text. The 60 words in the vocabulary list at the beginning of each chapter are pronounced and defined on these CDs.

- Caution: Do not limit your studying to these lists. Although they contain important terms, there are many additional words in each chapter that you need to know.

Use Your Flash Cards

- Use the flash cards from the back of this book.

- As you go through them, remove from the stack all the word parts you can define.

- Keep working until you have mastered all of the word parts.

Make Your Own Study List

- By now you should have greatly reduced the number of terms still to be mastered. Make a list of these terms and word parts, and concentrate on them.

Review Your Learning Exercises

As your corrected learning exercises are returned, save them. At review time go through these sheets and note where you made mistakes. Ask yourself, *"Do I know the correct answer now?"* If not, add the term or word part to your study list.

For the True/False questions in the learning exercises, you can challenge yourself to change all the "false" answers into true ones. For example, "Cholangiography is an endoscopic diagnostic procedure," is false. Ask yourself: "What is the correct definition of cholangiography?"

Help Someone Else

One of the greatest ways to really learn something is to teach it! If a classmate is having trouble, tutoring that person will help both of you learn the material.

Use the Practice Sessions

The next two pages are answer sheets to be used with the Review Session and Simulated Medical Terminology Final Test that follow.

REVIEW SESSION ANSWER SHEET

Write the **letter** of the correct answer on the line next to the question number.

RS.1. _____	RS.26. _____	RS.51. _____	RS.76. _____
RS.2. _____	RS.27. _____	RS.52. _____	RS.77. _____
RS.3. _____	RS.28. _____	RS.53. _____	RS.78. _____
RS.4. _____	RS.29. _____	RS.54. _____	RS.79. _____
RS.5. _____	RS.30. _____	RS.55. _____	RS.80. _____
RS.6. _____	RS.31. _____	RS.56. _____	RS.81. _____
RS.7. _____	RS.32. _____	RS.57. _____	RS.82. _____
RS.8. _____	RS.33. _____	RS.58. _____	RS.83. _____
RS.9. _____	RS.34. _____	RS.59. _____	RS.84. _____
RS.10. _____	RS.35. _____	RS.60. _____	RS.85. _____
RS.11. _____	RS.36. _____	RS.61. _____	RS.86. _____
RS.12. _____	RS.37. _____	RS.62. _____	RS.87. _____
RS.13. _____	RS.38. _____	RS.63. _____	RS.88. _____
RS.14. _____	RS.39. _____	RS.64. _____	RS.89. _____
RS.15. _____	RS.40. _____	RS.65. _____	RS.90. _____
RS.16. _____	RS.41. _____	RS.66. _____	RS.91. _____
RS.17. _____	RS.42. _____	RS.67. _____	RS.92. _____
RS.18. _____	RS.43. _____	RS.68. _____	RS.93. _____
RS.19. _____	RS.44. _____	RS.69. _____	RS.94. _____
RS.20. _____	RS.45. _____	RS.70. _____	RS.95. _____
RS.21. _____	RS.46. _____	RS.71. _____	RS.96. _____
RS.22. _____	RS.47. _____	RS.72. _____	RS.97. _____
RS.23. _____	RS.48. _____	RS.73. _____	RS.98. _____
RS.24. _____	RS.49. _____	RS.74. _____	RS.99. _____
RS.25. _____	RS.50. _____	RS.75. _____	RS.100. _____

Class _____   Name _____

SIMULATED MEDICAL TERMINOLOGY FINAL TEST ANSWER SHEET

Write the **letter** of the correct answer on the line next to the question number.

FT.1. _____	FT.26. _____	FT.51. _____	FT.76. _____
FT.2. _____	FT.27. _____	FT.52. _____	FT.77. _____
FT.3. _____	FT.28. _____	FT.53. _____	FT.78. _____
FT.4. _____	FT.29. _____	FT.54. _____	FT.79. _____
FT.5. _____	FT.30. _____	FT.55. _____	FT.80. _____
FT.6. _____	FT.31. _____	FT.56. _____	FT.81. _____
FT.7. _____	FT.32. _____	FT.57. _____	FT.82. _____
FT.8. _____	FT.33. _____	FT.58. _____	FT.83. _____
FT.9. _____	FT.34. _____	FT.59. _____	FT.84. _____
FT.10. _____	FT.35. _____	FT.60. _____	FT.85. _____
FT.11. _____	FT.36. _____	FT.61. _____	FT.86. _____
FT.12. _____	FT.37. _____	FT.62. _____	FT.87. _____
FT.13. _____	FT.38. _____	FT.63. _____	FT.88. _____
FT.14. _____	FT.39. _____	FT.64. _____	FT.89. _____
FT.15. _____	FT.40. _____	FT.65. _____	FT.90. _____
FT.16. _____	FT.41. _____	FT.66. _____	FT.91. _____
FT.17. _____	FT.42. _____	FT.67. _____	FT.92. _____
FT.18. _____	FT.43. _____	FT.68. _____	FT.93. _____
FT.19. _____	FT.44. _____	FT.69. _____	FT.94. _____
FT.20. _____	FT.45. _____	FT.70. _____	FT.95. _____
FT.21. _____	FT.46. _____	FT.71. _____	FT.96. _____
FT.22. _____	FT.47. _____	FT.72. _____	FT.97. _____
FT.23. _____	FT.48. _____	FT.73. _____	FT.98. _____
FT.24. _____	FT.49. _____	FT.74. _____	FT.99. _____
FT.25. _____	FT.50. _____	FT.75. _____	FT.100. _____

REVIEW SESSION

RS.1. An abnormally rapid rate of respiration usually of more than 20 breaths per minute is known as _____.

    a. bradypnea

    b. eupnea

    c. hyperventilation

    d. tachypnea

RS.2. An abnormally slow heart rate of less than 60 beats per minute is known as _____.

    a. atrial fibrillation

    b. bradycardia

    c. palpitation

    d. tachycardia

RS.3. The suffix _____ means surgical fixation.

    a. **-desis**

    b. **-lysis**

    c. **-pexy**

    d. **-ptosis**

RS.4. The presence of glucose in the urine is known as _____.

    a. albuminuria

    b. calciuria

    c. glycosuria

    d. hematuria

RS.5. A collection of pus within a body cavity is known as a/an _____.

    a. cyst

    b. empyema

    c. hernia

    d. tumor

RS.6. The grating sound heard when the ends of a broken bone move together is known as _____.

    a. closed reduction

    b. osteoclasis

    c. callus

    d. crepitation

RS.7. The abnormal development or growth of cells is known as _____.

    a. anaplasia

    b. dysplasia

    c. hyperplasia

    d. hypertrophy

RS.8. Which form of anemia is a genetic disorder?

    a. aplastic

    b. hemolytic

    c. megaloblastic

    d. sickle cell

RS.9. The processes through which the body maintains a constant internal environment are known as _____.

    a. hemothorax

    b. homeostasis

    c. hypophysis

    d. metabolism

RS.10. _____ is an inflammation of the myelin sheath of peripheral nerves, characterized by rapidly worsening muscle weakness that can lead to temporary paralysis.

    a. Bell's palsy

    b. Guillain-Barré syndrome

    c. Lou Gehrig's disease

    d. Raynaud's phenomenon

RS.11. The term _____ describes weakness or wearing away of body tissues and structures caused by pathology or by disuse of the muscle over a long period of time.

 a. adhesion

 b. ankylosis

 c. atrophy

 d. contracture

RS.12. The suffix _____ means blood or blood condition.

 a. **-emia**

 b. **-oma**

 c. **-pnea**

 d. **-uria**

RS.13. The procedure in which an anastomosis is created between the upper portion of the stomach and the duodenum is a/an _____.

 a. esophagogastrectomy

 b. esophagoplasty

 c. gastroduodenostomy

 d. gastrostomy

RS.14. Another term for conventional, or Western, medical practices and systems of health care is _____ medicine.

 a. alternative

 b. complementary

 c. allopathic

 d. integrative

RS.15. The term _____ means abnormal enlargement of the liver.

 a. hepatitis

 b. hepatomalacia

 c. hepatomegaly

 d. hepatorrhexis

RS.16. The term describing the prolapse of a kidney is _____.

 a. hydronephrosis

 b. nephroptosis

 c. nephropyosis

 d. nephropexy

RS.17. Which of these conditions is commonly known as a bruise?

 a. ecchymosis

 b. epistaxis

 c. hematoma

 d. lesion

RS.18. The acute respiratory infection known as _____ is characterized in children and infants by obstruction of the larynx, hoarseness, and a barking cough.

 a. asthma

 b. croup

 c. diphtheria

 d. pneumonia

RS.19. _____ is an autoimmune disease in which the body's own antibodies attack and destroy the cells of the thyroid gland.

 a. Conn's syndrome

 b. Hashimoto's disease

 c. Lou Gehrig's disease

 d. Graves' disease

RS.20. Which sexually transmitted disease can be detected through the VDRL blood test before the lesions appear?

 a. chlamydia

 b. gonorrhea

 c. syphilis

 d. trichomoniasis

RS.21. A blood clot attached to the interior wall of a vein or artery is known as a/an _____.

    a. embolism

    b. embolus

    c. thrombosis

    d. thrombus

RS.22. The term _____ describes the removal of a body part or the destruction of its function through the use of surgery, hormones, drugs, heat, chemicals, electrocautery, or other methods.

    a. ablation

    b. abrasion

    c. cryosurgery

    d. exfoliative cytology

RS.23. The term _____ describes any restriction to the opening of the mouth caused by trauma, surgery, or radiation associated with the treatment of oral cancer.

    a. atresia

    b. cachexia

    c. mastication

    d. trismus

RS.24. A woman who has borne one viable child is referred to as a _____

    a. nulligravida

    b. nullipara

    c. primigravida

    d. primipara

RS.25. The term _____ means inflammation of the pancreas.

    a. insulinoma

    b. pancreatectomy

    c. pancreatitis

    d. pancreatotomy

RS.26. The condition in which excess cerebrospinal fluid accumulates in the ventricles of the brain is known as _____.

    a. encephalocele

    b. hydrocephalus

    c. hydronephrosis

    d. hydroureter

RS.27. A _____ is the surgical fixation of a prolapsed vagina to a surrounding structure.

    a. colpopexy

    b. colporrhaphy

    c. cystopexy

    d. cystorrhaphy

RS.28. The combining form **metr/o** means _____.

    a. breast

    b. cervix

    c. menstruation

    d. uterus

RS.29. Which statement is accurate regarding cystic fibrosis (CF)?

    a. CF is a congenital disorder in which red blood cells take on a sickle shape.

    b. CF is also known as iron overload disease.

    c. CF is a genetic disorder that affects the lungs and digestive system.

    d. CF is characterized by short-lived red blood cells.

RS.30. The condition _____, which is thinner than average bone density, causes the patient to be at an increased risk of developing osteoporosis.

    a. osteochondroma

    b. osteopenia

    c. osteosclerosis

    d. rickets

RS.31. A/An _____ is a specialist who provides medical care to women during pregnancy, childbirth, and immediately thereafter.

    a. geriatrician

    b. gynecologist

    c. neonatologist

    d. obstetrician

RS.32. _____ is characterized by exophthalmos.

    a. Conn's syndrome

    b. Graves' disease

    c. Hashimoto's disease

    d. Huntington's disease

RS.33. The hormone _____ stimulates uterine contractions during childbirth.

    a. estrogen

    b. oxytocin

    c. progesterone

    d. testosterone

RS.34. A/An _____ is an unfavorable response due to prescribed medical treatment.

    a. idiopathic disorder

    b. nosocomial infection

    c. infectious disease

    d. iatrogenic illness

RS.35. The surgical freeing of a kidney from adhesions is known as _____.

    a. nephrolithiasis

    b. nephrolysis

    c. nephropyosis

    d. pyelitis

RS.36. _____ is the tissue death of an artery or arteries.

    a. arterionecrosis

    b. arteriostenosis

    c. atherosclerosis

    d. arthrosclerosis

RS.37. The _____ plane divides the body vertically into unequal left and right portions.

    a. frontal

    b. midsagittal

    c. sagittal

    d. transverse

RS.38. The term _____ means toward or nearer the midline.

    a. distal

    b. dorsal

    c. medial

    d. ventral

RS.39. A _____ was performed as a definitive test to determine if Alice Wilkinson has osteoporosis.

    a. bone marrow biopsy

    b. dual x-ray absorptiometry

    c. MRI

    d. nuclear bone scan

RS.40. The term _____ means movement of a limb away from the midline of the body.

    a. abduction

    b. adduction

    c. extension

    d. flexion

RS.41. When he fell, Manuel tore the posterior femoral muscles in his left leg. This is known as a/an _____ injury.

    a. Achilles tendon

    b. hamstring

    c. myofascial

    d. shin splint

RS.42. Mrs. Valladares has a bacterial infection of the lining of her heart. This condition is known as bacterial _____.

    a. endocarditis

    b. myocarditis

    c. pericarditis

    d. valvulitis

RS.43. The condition of _____ is commonly known as tooth decay.

    a. dental caries

    b. dental plaque

    c. gingivitis

    d. periodontal disease

RS.44. Henry was diagnosed as having an inflammation of the bone marrow and adjacent bone. Which term describes this condition?

    a. encephalitis

    b. meningitis

    c. osteomyelitis

    d. myelosis

RS.45. The term for an inflammation of the sheath surrounding a tendon is _____.

    a. bursitis

    b. tendinitis

    c. fasciitis

    d. tenosynovitis

RS.46. The term _____ describes drooping of the upper eyelid that is usually due to paralysis.

    a. ptosis

    b. dacryocystitis

    c. scleritis

    d. dacryoadenitis

RS.47. The combining form _____ means old age.

    a. **percuss/o**

    b. **presby/o**

    c. **prurit/o**

    d. **pseud/o**

RS.48. Mr. Ramirez had a heart attack. His physician recorded this as _____.

    a. angina

    b. a myocardial infarction

    c. congestive heart failure

    d. ischemic heart disease

RS.49. _____ is an abnormal increase in the number of red cells in the blood due to excess production of these cells by the bone marrow.

    a. anemia

    b. polycythemia

    c. thrombocytosis

    d. thrombocytopenia

RS.50. The common skin disorder _____ is characterized by flare-ups in which red papules covered with silvery scales occur on the elbows, knees, scalp, back, or buttocks.

    a. ichthyosis

    b. systemic lupus erythematosus

    c. psoriasis

    d. rosacea

RS.51. _____ is a group of disorders involving the parts of the brain that control thought, memory, and language.

   a. Alzheimer's disease

   b. catatonic behavior

   c. persistent vegetative state

   d. Reye's syndrome

RS.52. A/An _____ is a physician who specializes in physical medicine and rehabilitation with the focus on restoring function.

   a. exercise physiologist

   b. orthopedist

   c. physiatrist

   d. rheumatologist

RS.53. The term _____ describes a bone disorder of unknown cause that destroys normal bone structure and replaces it with fibrous tissue.

   a. costochondritis

   b. fibrous dysplasia

   c. osteomyelitis

   d. periostitis

RS.54. Slight paralysis of one side of the body is known as _____.

   a. hemiparesis

   b. hemiplegia

   c. myoparesis

   d. quadriplegia

RS.55. The _____ are the specialized cells that play an important role in blood clotting.

   a. basophils

   b. erythrocytes

   c. leukocytes

   d. thrombocytes

RS.56. The term _____ describes blood in the urine.

   a. hemangioma

   b. hematemesis

   c. hematoma

   d. hematuria

RS.57. The _____ receives the sound vibrations and relays them to the auditory nerve fibers.

   a. cochlea

   b. eustachian tube

   c. organ of Corti

   d. semicircular canal

RS.58. The _____ patrol the body, searching for antigens that produce infections. When such a cell is found, these cells grab, swallow, and internally break apart the captured antigen.

   a. B cells

   b. dendritic cells

   c. interleukins

   d. T cells

RS.59. The medical term for the congenital condition commonly known as clubfoot is _____.

   a. hallux valgus

   b. rickets

   c. spasmodic torticollis

   d. talipes

RS.60. A _____ is a normal scar resulting from the healing of a wound.

   a. callus

   b. cicatrix

   c. crepitus

   d. keloid

RS.61. The _____ is commonly known as the collar bone.

    a. clavicle

    b. olecranon

    c. patella

    d. sternum

RS.62. _____ are long, slender spiral-shaped bacteria that have flexible walls and are capable of movement.

    a. bacilli

    b. spirochetes

    c. staphylococcus

    d. streptococcus

RS.63. A/An _____ is a malignant tumor usually involving the upper shaft of long bones, the pelvis, or knee.

    a. adenocarcinoma

    b. Hodgkin's lymphoma

    c. osteochondroma

    d. osteosarcoma

RS.64. Which of these diseases is transmitted to humans by the bite of an infected blacklegged tick?

    a. cytomegalovirus

    b. human immunodeficiency virus

    c. Lyme disease

    d. West Nile virus

RS.65. _____ involves compression of nerves and blood vessels due to swelling within the enclosed space created by the fascia that separates groups of muscles.

    a. chronic fatigue syndrome

    b. compartment syndrome

    c. fibromyalgia syndrome

    d. myofascial pain syndrome

RS.66. A/An _____, also known as a *boil*, is a large, tender, swollen area caused by a staphylococcal infection around a hair follicle or sebaceous gland.

    a. abscess

    b. carbuncle

    c. furuncle

    d. pustule

RS.67. Which term refers to a class of drugs that relieves pain without affecting consciousness?

    a. analgesic

    b. barbiturate

    c. hypnotic

    d. sedative

RS.68. Fine muscle tremors, rigidity, and a slow or shuffling gait are all symptoms of the progressive condition known as _____.

    a. multiple sclerosis

    b. muscular dystrophy

    c. myasthenia gravis

    d. Parkinson's disease

RS.69. A form of vasculitis that affects the arms, upper body, neck, and head with symptoms including headache and touch sensitivity is known as _____.

    a. temporal arteritis

    b. hemangioma

    c. migraine

    d. peripheral vascular disease

RS.70. During her pregnancy, Ruth had a skin condition commonly known as the mask of pregnancy. The medical term for this condition is _____.

    a. chloasma

    b. albinism

    c. exanthem

    d. vitiligo

RS.71. _____ is caused by the failure of the bones of the limbs to grow to an appropriate length.

a. acromegaly

b. gigantism

c. hyperpituitarism

d. short stature

RS.72. In a _____ fracture, a bone is splintered or crushed.

a. comminuted

b. compound

c. compression

d. spiral

RS.73. The combining form _____ means vertebra or vertebral column.

a. **synovi/o**

b. **spondyl/o**

c. **scoli/o**

d. **splen/o**

RS.74. Which heart chamber receives oxygen-poor blood from all tissues, except the lungs?

a. left atrium

b. left ventricle

c. right atrium

d. right ventricle

RS.75. Which substance is commonly known as good cholesterol?

a. high-density lipoprotein cholesterol

b. homocysteine

c. low-density lipoprotein cholesterol

d. triglycerides

RS.76. Which symbol means less than?

a. >

b. ≥

c. <

d. i

RS.77. When medication is placed under the tongue and allowed to dissolve slowly, this is known as _____ administration.

a. oral

b. parenteral

c. sublingual

d. topical

RS.78. A sonogram is the image created by _____.

a. computerized tomography

b. fluoroscopy

c. magnetic resonance imaging (MRI)

d. ultrasonography

RS.79. Which combining form means red?

a. **melan/o**

b. **leuk/o**

c. **erythr/o**

d. **cyan/o**

RS.80. An autoimmune disorder characterized by a severe reaction to foods containing gluten is known as _____.

a. irritable bowel syndrome

b. diverticulosis

c. dyspepsia

d. celiac disease

RS.81. The term _____ describes inflammation of the gallbladder.

   a. cholecystectomy

   b. cholecystitis

   c. cholecystotomy

   d. cholelithiasis

RS.82. The term _____ means vomiting.

   a. emesis

   b. epistaxis

   c. reflux

   d. singultus

RS.83. The bluish discoloration of the skin caused by a lack of adequate oxygen is known as _____.

   a. cyanosis

   b. erythema

   c. jaundice

   d. pallor

RS.84. _____ is a disorder of the adrenal glands due to excessive production of aldosterone.

   a. Conn's syndrome

   b. Crohn's disease

   c. Cushing's syndrome

   d. Raynaud's phenomenon

RS.85. A/An _____ is any substance that the body regards as being foreign.

   a. allergen

   b. antibody

   c. antigen

   d. immunoglobulin

RS.86. Which condition has purple discolorations on the skin due to bleeding underneath the skin?

   a. dermatosis

   b. pruritus

   c. purpura

   d. suppuration

RS.87. A brief disturbance in brain function in which there is a loss of awareness often described as a staring episode is known as a/an _____ seizure.

   a. petit mal

   b. tonic-clonic

   c. absence

   d. grand mal

RS.88. A band of fibrous tissue that holds structures together abnormally is a/an _____.

   a. adhesion

   b. ankylosis

   c. contracture

   d. ligation

RS.89. Which procedure is performed to treat spider veins?

   a. blepharoplasty

   b. Botox

   c. liposuction

   d. sclerotherapy

RS.90. The instrument used to examine the external ear canal is known as a/an _____.

   a. anoscope

   b. ophthalmoscope

   c. otoscope

   d. speculum

RS.91. Which condition is breast cancer at its earliest stage before the cancer has broken through the wall of the milk duct?

   a. ductal carcinoma in situ

   b. infiltrating lobular carcinoma

   c. inflammatory breast cancer

   d. invasive lobular carcinoma

RS.92. Enlarged and swollen veins at the lower end of the esophagus are known as _____.

   a. esophageal aneurysms

   b. esophageal varices

   c. hemorrhoids

   d. varicose veins

RS.93. _____ is a progressive autoimmune disorder characterized by inflammation that causes demyelination of the myelin sheath.

   a. systemic lupus erythematosus

   b. multiple sclerosis

   c. muscular dystrophy

   d. spina bifida

RS.94. The abdominal region located below the stomach is known as the _____ region.

   a. epigastric

   b. hypogastric

   c. left hypochondriac

   d. umbilical

RS.95. Which of these sexually transmitted diseases is a bacterial infection?

   a. acquired immunodeficiency syndrome

   b. gonorrhea

   c. genital herpes

   d. trichomoniasis

RS.96. Narrowing of the opening of the foreskin so that it cannot be retracted to expose the glans penis is known as _____.

   a. balanitis

   b. Peyronie's disease

   c. phimosis

   d. priapism

RS.97. A/An _____ is an exfoliative screening biopsy for the detection and diagnosis of conditions of the cervix and surrounding tissues.

   a. endometrial biopsy

   b. lymph node dissection

   c. Pap smear

   d. sentinel node biopsy

RS.98. The term _____ is used to describe practices and systems of health care used to supplement traditional Western medicine.

   a. allopathic medicine

   b. complementary medicine

   c. alternative medicine

   d. homeopathy

RS.99. The term _____ describes turning the palm upward or forward.

   a. circumduction

   b. pronation

   c. rotation

   d. supination

RS.100. The term _____ describes the inflammation of a vein.

   a. vasculitis

   b. arteritis

   c. phlebitis

   d. phlebostenosis

SIMULATED FINAL TEST

FT.1. The term _____ describes a torn or jagged wound.

a. fissure

b. fistula

c. laceration

d. lesion

FT.2. The bone and soft tissues that surround and support the teeth are known as the _____.

a. dentition

b. rugae

c. gingiva

d. periodontium

FT.3. A chronic condition in which the heart is unable to pump out all of the blood that it receives is known as _____.

a. atrial fibrillation

b. heart failure

c. tachycardia

d. ventricular fibrillation

FT.4. Inflammation of the connective tissues that encloses the spinal cord and brain is known as _____.

a. encephalitis

b. encephalopathy

c. meningitis

d. myelopathy

FT.5. _____ is the partial or complete blockage of the small and/or large intestine that is caused by the stopping of normal intestinal peristalsis.

a. Crohn's disease

b. ileus

c. intussusception

d. intestinal obstruction

FT.6. The term _____ describes a condition in which the eye does not focus properly because of uneven curvatures of the cornea.

a. ametropia

b. astigmatism

c. ectropion

d. entropion

FT.7. A procedure in which pressurized fluid is used to clean out wound debris is known as _____.

a. irrigation and debridement

b. dilation and curettage

c. incision and drainage

d. dermabrasion

FT.8. The term _____ describes persistent severe burning pain that usually follows an injury to a sensory nerve.

a. causalgia

b. hyperesthesia

c. paresthesia

d. peripheral neuropathy

FT.9. A/An _____ is performed to reduce the risk of a stroke caused by a disruption of the blood flow to the brain.

a. aneurysmectomy

b. arteriectomy

c. carotid endarterectomy

d. coronary artery bypass graft

FT. 10. The term _____ means bleeding from the ear.

a. barotrauma

b. otomycosis

c. otopyorrhea

d. otorrhagia

FT.11. The medical term meaning itching is _____.

a. perfusion

b. pruritus

c. purpura

d. suppuration

FT.12. _____ is a condition characterized by episodes of severe chest pain due to inadequate blood flow to the myocardium.

a. angina

b. claudication

c. cyanosis

d. myocardial infarction

FT.13. The greenish material that forms the first stools of a newborn is known as _____.

a. colostrum

b. lochia

c. meconium

d. vernix

FT.14. A/An _____ is the result of medical treatment that yields the exact opposite of normally expected results.

a. drug interaction

b. paradoxical reaction

c. placebo

d. idiosyncratic reaction

FT.15. A _____ is a prediction of the probable course and outcome of a disease or disorder.

a. differential diagnosis

b. diagnosis

c. prognosis

d. syndrome

FT.16. _____ is a yellow discoloration of the skin, mucous membranes, and the eyes.

a. vitiligo

b. jaundice

c. erythema

d. albinism

FT.17. A/An _____ occurs at the lower end of the radius when a person tries to break a fall by landing on his or her hands.

a. Colles' fracture

b. comminuted fracture

c. osteoporotic hip fracture

d. spiral fracture

FT.18. The term _____ describes excessive urination during the night.

a. nocturia

b. polydipsia

c. polyuria

d. urinary retention

FT.19. A closed sac associated with a sebaceous gland that contains yellow, fatty material is known as a _____.

   a. comedo

   b. sebaceous cyst

   c. seborrheic dermatitis

   d. seborrheic keratosis

FT.20. The term _____ describes the condition commonly known as swollen glands.

   a. adenoiditis

   b. vasculitis

   c. lymphadenitis

   d. lymphangioma

FT.21. A/An _____ is a sudden, involuntary contraction of one or more muscles.

   a. adhesion

   b. contracture

   c. spasm

   d. sprain

FT.22. _____ is the respiratory disease commonly known as whooping cough.

   a. croup

   b. diphtheria

   c. emphysema

   d. pertussis

FT.23. The lymphocytes that play an important role in the killing of cancer cells and cells infected by viruses are known as _____.

   a. cytokines

   b. natural killer cells

   c. B cells

   d. T cells

FT.24. _____ is an abnormal lateral curvature of the spine.

   a. kyphosis

   b. lordosis

   c. lumbago

   d. scoliosis

FT.25. The surgical creation of an artificial excretory opening between the ileum and the outside of the abdominal wall is a/an _____.

   a. colostomy

   b. enteropexy

   c. gastroptosis

   d. ileostomy

FT.26. Which examination technique is the visualization of body parts in motion by projecting x-ray images on a luminous fluorescent screen?

   a. computed tomography

   b. fluoroscopy

   c. magnetic resonance imaging

   d. radiography

FT.27. As the condition known as _____ progresses, the chest sometimes assumes an enlarged barrel shape.

   a. asthma

   b. diphtheria

   c. emphysema

   d. epistaxis

FT.28. The term _____ means to stop or control bleeding.

   a. hemorrhage

   b. hemostasis

   c. homeostasis

   d. thrombocytopenia

FT.29. An accumulation of pus in the fallopian tube is known as _____.

  a. leukorrhea

  b. otopyorrhea

  c. pyosalpinx

  d. salpingitis

FT.30. A _____ is the bruising of brain tissue as a result of a head injury.

  a. cerebral contusion

  b. concussion

  c. hydrocele

  d. meningocele

FT.31. The term _____ means vomiting blood.

  a. epistaxis

  b. hemarthrosis

  c. hematemesis

  d. hyperemesis

FT.32. _____ is a diagnostic procedure designed to determine the density of a body part by the sound produced by tapping the surface with the fingers.

  a. auscultation

  b. palpation

  c. percussion

  d. range of motion

FT.33. Abnormally rapid, deep breathing resulting in decreased levels of carbon dioxide in the blood is known as _____.

  a. apnea

  b. dyspnea

  c. hyperventilation

  d. hypoventilation

FT.34. The term _____ describes difficult or painful urination.

  a. dyspepsia

  b. dysphagia

  c. dystrophy

  d. dysuria

FT.35. A _____ is a false personal belief that is maintained despite obvious proof or evidence to the contrary.

  a. delusion

  b. dementia

  c. mania

  d. phobia

FT.36. In _____, the normal rhythmic contractions of the atria are replaced by rapid irregular twitching of the muscular heart wall.

  a. atrial fibrillation

  b. bradycardia

  c. tachycardia

  d. ventricular fibrillation

FT.37. The eye condition known as _____ is characterized by increased intraocular pressure.

  a. cataracts

  b. glaucoma

  c. macular degeneration

  d. monochromatism

FT.38. _____ is the presence of blood in the seminal fluid.

  a. azoospermia

  b. hematuria

  c. hematospermia

  d. prostatorrhea

FT.39. The condition of common changes in the eyes that occur with aging is known as _____.

    a. hyperopia

    b. presbycusis

    c. presbyopia

    d. strabismus

FT.40. Which body cavity protects the brain?

    a. anterior

    b. cranial

    c. caudal

    d. ventral

FT.41. A hernia of the bladder through the vaginal wall is known as a _____.

    a. cystocele

    b. cystopexy

    c. vaginocele

    d. vesicovaginal fistula

FT.42. Which condition of a young child is characterized by the inability to develop normal social relationships?

    a. autism

    b. attention deficit disorder

    c. dyslexia

    d. mental retardation

FT.43. A ringing, buzzing, or roaring sound in one or both ears is known as _____.

    a. labyrinthitis

    b. syncope

    c. tinnitus

    d. vertigo

FT.44. A/An _____ is an outbreak of a disease occurring over a large geographic area that is possibly worldwide.

    a. endemic

    b. epidemic

    c. pandemic

    d. syndrome

FT.45. _____ is an abnormal accumulation of serous fluid in the peritoneal cavity.

    a. ascites

    b. aerophagia

    c. melena

    d. bolus

FT.46. A _____ is a discolored flat spot that is less than 1 cm in diameter, such as a freckle.

    a. macule

    b. papule

    c. plaque

    d. vesicle

FT.47. The western blot test is used to _____.

    a. confirm an HIV infection

    b. detect hepatitis C

    c. diagnose Kaposi's sarcoma

    d. test for tuberculosis

FT.48. The term _____ describes excessive uterine bleeding at both the usual time of menstrual periods and at other irregular intervals.

    a. dysmenorrhea

    b. hypermenorrhea

    c. menometrorrhagia

    d. oligomenorrhea

FT.49. _____is a form of sexual dysfunction in which the penis is bent or curved during erection.

a. erectile dysfunction

b. Peyronie's disease

c. phimosis

d. priapism

FT.50. A/An _____ is an abnormal sound or murmur heard during auscultation of an artery.

a. auscultation

b. bruit

c. rhonchi

d. stridor

FT.51. The condition commonly known as wear-and-tear arthritis is _____.

a. gouty arthritis

b. osteoarthritis

c. rheumatoid arthritis

d. spondylosis

FT.52. The term _____ means to free a tendon from adhesions.

a. tenodesis

b. tenolysis

c. tenorrhaphy

d. insertion

FT.53. The malignant condition known as _____ is distinguished by the presence of Reed-Sternberg cells.

a. Hodgkin's lymphoma

b. leukemia

c. non-Hodgkin's lymphoma

d. osteosarcoma

FT.54. The chronic, degenerative disease characterized by scarring that causes disturbance of the structure and function of the liver is _____.

a. cirrhosis

b. hepatitis

c. hepatomegaly

d. jaundice

FT.55. _____ removes waste products directly from the bloodstream of patients whose kidneys no longer function.

a. diuresis

b. epispadias

c. hemodialysis

d. peritoneal dialysis

FT.56. The medical term for the condition commonly known as fainting is _____.

a. comatose

b. singultus

c. stupor

d. syncope

FT.57. _____is a condition in which there is an insufficient supply of oxygen in the tissues due to a restricted blood flow to a part of the body.

a. angina

b. infarction

c. ischemia

d. perfusion

FT.58. A collection of blood in the pleural cavity is known as a _____.

a. hemophilia

b. hemoptysis

c. hemostasis

d. hemothorax

FT.59. The return of swallowed food
into the mouth is known as
_____.

    a. dysphagia

    b. emesis

    c. pyrosis

    d. regurgitation

FT.60. An inflammation of the lacrimal gland
that could be caused by a bacterial,
viral, or fungal infection is known as
_____.

    a. anisocoria

    b. dacryoadenitis

    c. exophthalmos

    d. hordeolum

FT.61. The contraction of the pupil, normally
in response to exposure to light,
but also possibly due to the use of
prescription or illegal drugs, is known as
_____.

    a. nystagmus

    b. mydriasis

    c. miosis

    d. mycosis

FT.62. The term _____ means
excessive urination.

    a. enuresis

    b. oliguria

    c. overactive bladder

    d. polyuria

FT.63. The surgical removal of the gallbladder is
known as a _____.

    a. cholecystectomy

    b. cholecystostomy

    c. cholecystotomy

    d. choledocholithotomy

FT.64. An elevated _____
indicates the presence of inflammation in
the body.

    a. complete blood cell count

    b. erythrocyte sedimentation rate

    c. platelet count

    d. total hemoglobin test

FT.65. A/An _____ is a groove
or cracklike break in the skin.

    a. abrasion

    b. fissure

    c. laceration

    d. ulcer

FT.66. A/An _____ injection
is made into the fatty layer just below the
skin.

    a. intradermal

    b. intramuscular

    c. intravenous

    d. subcutaneous

FT.67. The _____ has roles in
both the immune and endocrine systems.

    a. pancreas

    b. pituitary

    c. spleen

    d. thymus

FT.68. The medical term
_____ describes an
inflammation of the brain.

    a. encephalitis

    b. mastitis

    c. meningitis

    d. myelitis

FT.69. The hormone secreted by fat cells is known as _____.

    a. interstitial cell-stimulating hormone

    b. growth hormone

    c. leptin

    d. neurohormone

FT.70. A type of catheter made of a flexible tube with a balloon filled with sterile water at the end to hold it in place in the bladder is known as a _____ catheter.

    a. Foley

    b. indwelling

    c. suprapubic

    d. intermittent

FT.71. A/An _____ is acquired in a hospital or clinic setting.

    a. functional disorder

    b. iatrogenic illness

    c. idiopathic disorder

    d. nosocomial infection

FT.72. A type of pneumonia contracted during a stay in the hospital when the patient's defenses are impaired is known as _____ pneumonia.

    a. hospital-acquired

    b. aspiration

    c. community-acquired

    d. walking

FT.73. The term _____ describes an eye disorder that can develop as a complication of diabetes.

    a. diabetic neuropathy

    b. diabetic retinopathy

    c. papilledema

    d. retinal detachment

FT.74. The physical wasting with the loss of weight and muscle mass due to diseases such as advanced cancer is known as _____.

    a. cachexia

    b. anorexia nervosa

    c. bulimia nervosa

    d. malnutrition

FT.75. The term _____ means difficulty in swallowing.

    a. aerophagia

    b. dyspepsia

    c. dysphagia

    d. eructation

FT.76. A/An _____ occurs when a blood vessel in the brain leaks or ruptures.

    a. cerebral hematoma

    b. embolism

    c. hemorrhagic stroke

    d. ischemic stroke

FT.77. The hormonal disorder known as _____ results from the pituitary gland producing too much growth hormone in adults.

    a. acromegaly

    b. cretinism

    c. gigantism

    d. pituitarism

FT.78. The term _____ describes the condition commonly known an ingrown toenail.

    a. cryptorchidism

    b. onychocryptosis

    c. onychomycosis

    d. priapism

FT.79. An _____ is the instrument used to examine the interior of the eye.

a. ophtalmoscope

b. ophthalmoscope

c. opthalmoscope

d. opthlmoscope

FT.80. A/An _____ is a protrusion of part of the stomach upward into the chest through an opening in the diaphragm.

a. esophageal hernia

b. esophageal varices

c. hiatal hernia

d. hiatal varices

FT.81. An _____ is a surgical incision made to enlarge the vaginal orifice to facilitate childbirth.

a. episiorrhaphy

b. episiotomy

c. epispadias

d. epistaxis

FT.82. Severe itching of the external female genitalia is known as _____.

a. colpitis

b. leukorrhea

c. pruritus vulvae

d. vaginal candidiasis

FT.83. _____ is a urinary problem caused by interference with the normal nerve pathways associated with urination.

a. neurogenic bladder

b. overactive bladder

c. polyuria

d. overflow incontinence

FT.84. A/An _____ is an instrument used to enlarge the opening of any canal or cavity to facilitate inspection of its interior.

a. endoscope

b. speculum

c. sphygmomanometer

d. stethoscope

FT.85. A _____, also known as *scab*, is a collection of dried serum and cellular debris.

a. crust

b. nodule

c. plaque

d. scale

FT.86. A _____ is a type of cancer that occurs in blood-making cells found in the red bone marrow.

a. carcinoma

b. myeloma

c. osteochondroma

d. sarcoma

FT.87. _____ can occur when a foreign substance, such as vomit, is inhaled into the lungs.

a. aspiration pneumonia

b. bacterial pneumonia

c. walking pneumonia

d. Pneumocystis pneumonia

FT.88. The condition known as _____ is ankylosis of the bones of the middle ear that causes a conductive hearing loss.

a. labyrinthitis

b. mastoiditis

c. osteosclerosis

d. otosclerosis

FT.89. The procedure known as _____ is the surgical fusion of two bones to stiffen a joint.

    a. arthrodesis

    b. arthrolysis

    c. synovectomy

    d. tenodesis

FT.90. The suffix _____ means rupture.

    a. **-rrhage**

    b. **-rrhaphy**

    c. **-rrhea**

    d. **-rrhexis**

FT.91. An abnormal fear of being in small or enclosed spaces is known as _____.

    a. acrophobia

    b. agoraphobia

    c. social phobia

    d. claustrophobia

FT.92. _____ is the distortion or impairment of voluntary movement such as in a tic or spasm.

    a. bradykinesia

    b. dyskinesia

    c. hyperkinesia

    d. myoclonus

FT.93. Which structure secretes bile?

    a. gallbladder

    b. liver

    c. pancreas

    d. spleen

FT.94. _____ is the process of recording the electrical activity of the brain.

    a. echoencephalograph

    b. electroencephalography

    c. electromyography

    d. magnetic resonance imaging

FT.95. The suffix _____ means surgical fixation.

    a. **-lysis**

    b. **-rrhaphy**

    c. **-desis**

    d. **-pexy**

FT.96. The eye condition that causes the loss of central vision, but not total blindness, is known as _____.

    a. cataracts

    b. glaucoma

    c. macular degeneration

    d. presbyopia

FT.97. A/An _____ is performed to remove excess skin and fat for the elimination of wrinkles.

    a. ablation

    b. blepharoplasty

    c. rhytidectomy

    d. sclerotherapy

FT.98. The condition known as _____ describes total paralysis affecting only one side of the body.

    a. hemiparesis

    b. hemiplegia

    c. paraplegia

    d. quadriplegia

FT.99. _____ is a new cancer site that results from the spreading process.

   a. in situ

   b. metabolism

   c. metastasis

   d. metastasize

FT.100. Which of these hormones is produced by the pituitary gland?

   a. adrenocorticotropic hormone

   b. calcitonin

   c. cortisol

   d. epinephrine

NOTES

NOTES

INSTRUCTIONS

- Carefully remove the flash card pages from the workbook, and separate them to create 160 flash cards.

- There are three types of cards: **prefixes** (such as **a-** and **hyper-**), **suffixes** (such as **-graphy** and **-rrhagia**), and **word roots/combining forms** (such as **gastr/o** and **arthr/o**). All of the cards have the definition on the back. Prefixes and suffixes also have the type of word part listed on the front of each card.

- The word root/combining form cards are arranged by body systems. This allows you to sort out the cards you want to study based on where you are in the book. Use the "general" cards throughout your course.

- Use the flash cards to memorize word parts, to test yourself, and for periodic review.

- By putting cards together, you can create terms just as you did in the challenge word building exercises.

- You can create flash cards for word parts that are not already included by using the page of blank cards at the back. For additional cards, we recommend sheets of perforated business card stock available at any office supply store.

WORD PART GAMES

Here are games you can play with one or more partners to help you learn word parts using your flash cards.

The Review Game

Word Parts Up: Shuffle the deck of flash cards. Put the pile, *word parts up*, in the center of the desk. Take turns choosing a card from anywhere in the deck and giving the definition of the word part shown. If you get it right, you get to keep it. If you miss, it goes into the discard pile. When the draw pile is gone, whoever has the largest pile wins.

Definitions Up: Shuffle the deck of flash cards and place them with the *definition side up*. Play the review game the same way.

The Create-a-Word Game

Shuffle the deck and deal each person 14 cards, *word parts up*. Place the remaining draw pile in the center of the desk, *word parts down*.

Each player should try to create as many legitimate medical words as possible using the cards he or she has been dealt. Then take turns discarding one card (word part up, in the discard pile) and taking one. When it is your turn to discard a card, you may choose either the card the previous player discarded or a "mystery card" from the draw pile. Continue working on words until all the cards in the draw pile have been taken.

To score, each player must define every word created correctly. If the definition is correct, the player receives one point for each card used. If it is incorrect, two points are deducted for each card in that word. Unused cards count as one point off each. Whoever has the highest number of points wins. Note: Use your medical dictionary or a recognized online resource if there is any doubt that a word is legitimate!

prefix

A-, AN-

prefix

END-, ENDO-

prefix

ANTE-

prefix

HEMI-

prefix

ANTI-

prefix

HYPER-

prefix

BRADY-

prefix

HYPO-

prefix

DYS-

prefix

INTER-

within, in, inside

without, away from,
negative, not

half

before, in front of, forward

excessive, increased

against

deficient, decreased

slow

between, among

bad, difficult, painful

prefix

INTRA-

prefix

POST-

prefix

NEO-

prefix

PRE-

prefix

PER-

prefix

SUB-

prefix

PERI-

prefix

SUPER-, SUPRA-

prefix

POLY-

prefix

TACHY-

after, behind

within, inside

before, in front of, forward

new, strange

under, less, below

excessive, through

above, excessive

surrounding, around

fast, rapid

many

suffix

-AC, -AL

suffix

-CYTE

suffix

-ALGIA

suffix

-DESIS

suffix

-ARY

suffix

-ECTOMY

suffix

-CELE

suffix

-ECTASIS

suffix

-CENTESIS

suffix

-EMIA

cell

pertaining to, relating to

to bind, tie together

pain, suffering, painful condition

surgical removal, cutting out

pertaining to

stretching, dilation, enlargement

hernia, tumor, swelling

blood, blood condition

surgical puncture to remove fluid

suffix

-ESTHESIA

suffix

-ITIS

suffix

-GRAM, -GRAPH

suffix

-LYSIS

suffix

-GRAPHY

suffix

-MALACIA

suffix

-IA

suffix

-MEGALY

suffix

-IC

suffix

-NECROSIS

inflammation

sensation, feeling

breakdown, separation,
setting free, destruction,
loosening

a picture or record

abnormal softening

the process of producing a
picture or record

enlargement

abnormal condition,
disease

tissue death

pertaining to

suffix

-OLOGIST

suffix

-OTOMY

suffix

-OLOGY

suffix

-PATHY

suffix

-OMA

suffix

-PAUSE

suffix

-OSIS

suffix

-PEXY

suffix

-OSTOMY

suffix

-PLASTY

cutting, surgical incision

specialist

disease, suffering,
feeling, emotion

the science or study of

stopping

tumor, neoplasm

surgical fixation

abnormal condition,
disease

surgical repair

surgical creation of an
opening to the body surface

suffix

-PLEGIA

suffix

-RRHEA

suffix

-PNEA

suffix

-RRHEXIS

suffix

-PTOSIS

suffix

-SCLEROSIS

suffix

-RRHAGIA, -RRHAGE

suffix

-SCOPE

suffix

-RRHAPHY

suffix

-SCOPY

flow or discharge

paralysis

rupture

breathing

abnormal hardening

prolapse, drooping forward

instrument for visual
examination

bleeding, abnormal
excessive fluid discharge

visual examination

surgical suturing

suffix

-STENOSIS

Cardiovascular System

ARTERI/O

suffix

-TRIPSY

Cardiovascular System

ATHER/O

suffix

-URIA

Cardiovascular System

**CARD/O,
CARDI/O**

Cardiovascular System

ANGI/O

Cardiovascular System

**HEM/O,
HEMAT/O**

Cardiovascular System

AORT/O

Cardiovascular System

PHLEB/O

artery

abnormal narrowing

plaque, fatty substance

to crush

heart

urination, urine

blood, pertaining to the blood

pertaining to blood or lymph vessels

vein

aorta

Cardiovascular System

THROMB/O

Digestive System

COL/O, COLON/O

Cardiovascular System

VEN/O

Digestive System

PROCT/O

Diagnostic Procedures

ECH/O

Digestive System

ENTER/O

Diagnostic Procedures

RADI/O

Digestive System

ESOPHAG/O

Digestive System

CHOLECYST/O

Digestive System

GASTR/O

colon, large intestine

clot

anus and rectum

vein

small intestine

sound

esophagus

radiation, x-rays

stomach

gallbladder

Digestive System

HEPAT/O

Endocrine System

THYR/O, THYROID/O

Digestive System

SIGMOID/O

General

ADIP/O

Endocrine System

ADREN/O

General

ALBIN/O

Endocrine & Reproductive Systems

GONAD/O

General

CEPHAL/O

Endocrine & Digestive Systems

PANCREAT/O

General

CERVIC/O

thyroid gland

liver

fat

sigmoid colon

white

adrenal glands

head

sex gland

neck, cervix

pancreas

CORON/O

LAPAR/O

CYAN/O

LEUK/O

CYT/O

LIP/O

ERYTHR/O

MELAN/O

HIST/O

MYC/O

abdomen,
abdominal wall

coronary, crown

white

blue

fat, lipid

cell

black, dark

red

fungus

tissue

General

PATH/O

Immune System

ONC/O

General

PY/O

Integumentary System

CUTANE/O

General

PYR/O

Integumentary System

DERM/O, DERMAT/O

General

SARC/O

Integumentary System

HIDR/O

Immune System

CARCIN/O

Integumentary System

SEB/O

tumor

disease, suffering,
feeling, emotion

skin

pus

skin

fever, fire

sweat

flesh, connective tissue

sebum

cancerous

Integumentary System

UNGU/O

Muscular System

MY/O

Integumentary System

XER/O

Muscular System

TEN/O, TEND/O, TENDIN/O

General

ADEN/O

Nervous System

ENCEPHAL/O

Lymphatic System

SPLEN/O

Nervous System

MENING/O

Muscular System

FASCI/O

Nervous System

NEUR/I, NEUR/O

muscle

nail

tendon, stretch out, extend, strain

dry

brain

gland

meninges, membranes

spleen

nerve, nerve tissue

fascia, fibrous band

Reproductive Systems

COLP/O

Reproductive Systems

OOPHOR/O, OVARI/O

Reproductive Systems

HYSTER/O

Reproductive Systems

ORCH/O, ORCHID/O

Reproductive Systems

MEN/O

Reproductive Systems & Special Senses

SALPING/O

Reproductive Systems

METR/O, METRI/O, METR/I

Reproductive Systems

UTER/O

Reproductive Systems

OV/O

Reproductive Systems

VAGIN/O

ovary

vagina

testicles, testis, testes

uterus

uterine (fallopian) tube,
auditory (eustachian) tube

menstruation, menses

uterus

uterus

vagina

egg

Respiratory System

BRONCH/O, BRONCHI/O

Respiratory System

PULM/O, PULMON/O

Respiratory System

LARYNG/O

Respiratory System

TRACHE/O

Respiratory System

PHARYNG/O

Skeletal System

ANKYL/O

Respiratory System

PLEUR/O

Skeletal System

ARTHR/O

Respiratory System

PNEUM/O, PNEUMON/O

Skeletal System

CHONDR/O

lung

bronchial tube, bronchus

trachea, windpipe

larynx, throat

crooked, bent, stiff

throat, pharynx

joint

pleura, side of the body

cartilage

lung, air

Skeletal System

COST/O

Skeletal & Respiratory Systems

THORAC/O

Skeletal System

CRANI/O

Special Senses & Integumentary System

KERAT/O

Skeletal & Nervous System

MYEL/O

Special Senses

MYRING/O

Skeletal System

OSS/E, OSS/I, OST/O, OSTE/O

Special Senses

OPTIC/O, OPT/O

Skeletal System

SPONDYL/O

Special Senses

OT/O

chest

rib

horny, hard, cornea

skull

tympanic membrane,
eardrum

spinal cord, bone marrow

eye, vision

bone

ear, hearing

vertebrae, vertebral
column, backbone

Special Senses

RETIN/O

Urinary System

NEPHR/O

**Special Senses &
Integumentary System**

SCLER/O

Urinary System

PYEL/O

Special Senses

TYMPAN/O

Urinary System

REN/O

Urinary System

CYST/O

Urinary System

URETER/O

Urinary & Digestive System

LITH/O

Urinary System

URETHR/O

kidney

retina

renal pelvis, bowl of kidney

sclera, white of eye, hard

kidney

tympanic membrane,
eardrum

ureter

urinary bladder, cyst, sac
of fluid

urethra

stone, calculus